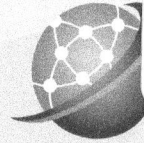

Prep Your Way
Workshops | Online Courses | Workbooks

Associate Safety Professional (ASP)	**Certified Instructional Trainer (CIT)**	**Certified Hazardous Materials Manager (CHMM)**
Construction Health and Safety Technician (CHST)	**Certified Industrial Hygienist (CIH)**	**Certified Safety Professional (CSP)**
Occupational Hygiene and Safety Technologist (OHST)	**Safety Management Specialist (SMS)**	**Safety Trained Supervisor (STS)**

Safety Trained Supervisor Construction (STSC)

SPAN™ **Exam Prep** is the leading certification exam study solution to prepare safety professionals for exams from the Board of Certified Safety Professionals (BCSP). This BCSP exam prep helps professionals achieve important career goals through advancing competencies for safety management excellence. As the leader in BCSP exam preparation since 1992, SPAN offers live workshops, online courses and workbooks. The self-directed study materials are designed for professionals looking to gain critical knowledge, study techniques, and testing strategies to pass certification examinations.

www.spansafety.com

CHST Exam Study Workbook Volume I

Dedicated to All Safety, Health and Environmental Professionals

Striving to Protect

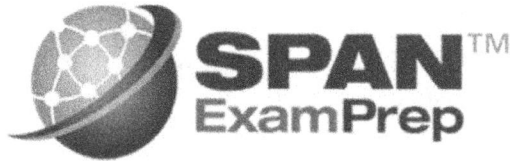

SPAN™ ExamPrep

www.spansafety.com

This Publication is not intended to guarantee that the user will pass an exam, become certified or in general may not cover every aspect of the certification process.

The information contained in this study workbook is intended to be used in preparation for the Construction Health and Safety Technologist® examination and should not be used as an authority in the professional practice of safety, health, or environmental compliance.

The Construction Health and Safety Technologist® (CHST®) Certification is a registered trademark of the Board of Certified Safety Professionals (BCSP). The opinions expressed are those of the authors and no guarantee, warranty, or other representation is made as to the absolute correctness or sufficiency of any information contained in this study workbook.

Daniel J. Snyder, Ed.D, CSP, CHST
Copyright © 2019 by SPAN™ International Training, LLC
402 W. Mt Vernon St #111
Nixa, Missouri 65714
Phone: 417 724 8348
info@spansafetyworkshops.com

ISBN 978-1-891017-70-4 (set)
ISBN 978-1-891017-68-1 (v.1)
ISBN 978-1-891017-69-8 (v.2)

Contents

Introduction

There are two primary goals of this professional development course (PDC):

1. Provide candidates the knowledge and skills to successfully attain Construction Health and Safety Technologist® (CHST®) certification.

2. Enhance skills, knowledge and abilities as a safety professional.

This workbook is designed to be used as a resource for self-directed study in preparation for the CHST exam. In the fast track three-day workshop conducted by SPAN™ International Training, LLC, participants are provided expert guidance and use the same content presented in these workbooks. This curriculum is also used in the online SPAN™ CertBoK® Exam Learning Management System (LMS).

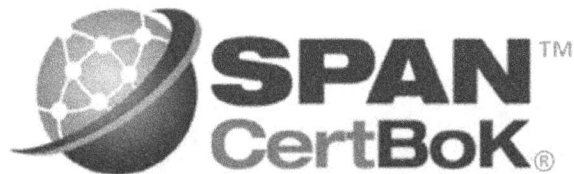

Workshops are conducted periodically throughout the year so that professionals can take the examination as soon as they are prepared. Visit the SPAN website for workshop dates and locations. www.spansafety.com

The exam is designed for candidates with 1 year of professional safety experience with a high school diploma or GED, and 3 years' experience with 35% of professional duties are dedicated to safety and health. Generally, it takes the average safety and health practitioner about 40-100 hours of dedicated self-study, in addition to a workshop, to adequately prepare for the examination. The self-study can generally be accomplished in about 4 to 12 weeks depending on individual needs.

The workbook is divided into two volumes designed for self-study and facilitated professional development workshops. After each section of the workbook there are fully developed explanations for the answer selected for each question. In many cases information about all the selections offered as possible answers will be included to assist in developing a better understanding of the subject. Each section is designed to allow the safety professional to measure progress during the extended program of self-study that is normally required to pass the CHST certification exam.

Considerable effort has been made to fully develop and explain the concepts and techniques discussed. However, given the differences in the background and experience of the safety practitioners sitting for the CHST examination, it is impossible to explain all concepts to all candidates. The materials are based on the exam blueprint and subject matter expertise.

After reviewing the workbook, you should identify your individual knowledge gaps and establish a study plan. There are voluminous resources available for each domain of the exam blueprint. Simply stated, chance favors the prepared mind and candidates should have a study plan. Budget adequate time to master the material.

This workbook is designed to optimize study time. There is no extraneous or "nice to know" information in this workbook. All the information is important. Concentrating on the areas emphasized in the text should reduce research and study time considerably.

The BCSP exams change regularly, usually on a 5-year cycle to reflect the contemporary state of the profession. SPAN™ conducts ongoing research and development to ensure the accuracy and quality of the curriculum based on the actual exam blueprint. ***This workbook does not contain actual CHST test questions.*** The curriculum is designed using a multiple-choice question and answer learning format with detailed explanations that are representative of competencies reflected in the blueprint and on the exam. Concepts and content are paraphrased format to allow broad coverage of the material and optimize your study efforts.

The beginning sections of the workbook are devoted to enhancing knowledge and skills in:
- The exam process
- Study and testing techniques
- Applied Math and Science problems

The content is designed to engage the analytical portions of the brain and help prepare you for the mathematical components of the exam.

From the introductory and math review sections, the workbook progresses to individual areas on each of the seven CHST exam blueprint domains. These seven blueprint domains utilize the question and answer format designed to mimic the type of questions offered on the exam. Explanations are offered to reduce research time considering the examination covers a tremendous amount of subject matter.

The questions presented are representative of the questions found on the actual examination. For this reason, you must gain enough knowledge the area (areas) to which the question is pertaining, which may require additional study.

Approximately 67% of the scored questions must be answered correctly to pass the CHST examination. Repetition will help you identify areas of strength and weakness and close the knowledge gaps.

The assumption is made that only fully qualified safety practitioners will attempt to sit for the CHST examination, which means everyone using this workbook has a fundamental knowledge in the Safety and Health field. Given this assumption, no attempt has been made to provide a comprehensive safety text. The workbook is designed as a guide and depending upon an individual's knowledge baseline, additional research may be required.

The challenge of achieving certification is a difficult task. Embrace the journey of professional development in preparation for the exam. The modern safety professional must be a dynamic adaptive leader and lifelong learner.

This curriculum has been carefully checked for accuracy, but errors may exist. Should and an error be discovered, contact the author via info@spansafetyworkshops.com

BCSP Certification Matrix

	CSP	ASP	GSP	SMS	OHST	CHST3	STS/ STSC	CET
Minimum Education	Bachelor's degree [1] or Associate's degree [2]	Bachelor's degree or Associate's degree	Bachelor's or Master's degree [3]	High School Diploma or GED	High School Diploma or GED	High School Diploma or GED	N/A	High School Diploma or GED
Minimum Training	N/A [4]	N/A	N/A	N/A	N/A	N/A	30 hours of SH&E [5] training	Delivery of 135 hours of training [6]
Minimum Work Experience	4 years of experience [7] And Hold an authorized credential [8]	1 year of experience [9]	No experience required [10]	10 years of safety management related experience [11]	3 years of experience [12]	3 years of construction experience [13]	2 years supervisory experience [14] Or 4 years' work experience	Hold an authorized credential [15]
Application Fees	$160	$160	N/A	$160	$140	$140	$120	$140
Examination Fees	$350	$350	N/A	$350	$300	$300	$185	$300
Eligibility Extension Fees	$100	$100	N/A	$100	$100	$100	$100	$100
Renewal Fees	$150	$140	$140	$140	$120	$120	$60	$120
Passing Scores	100/175 57%	107/175 61%	N/A	106/175 60.5%	116/175 66.2%	108/175 61.7%	STS: 61/87 70.1% STSC: 60/87 68.9%	119/175 68%
Recertification (5-year cycle)	25 points	25 points	N/A	25 points	20 points	20 points	30 hours of safety and health courses [16]	20 points [17]

[1] In any field

[2] In a safety and health or related field

[3] from an ABETASAC or AABI accredited QAP program

[4] Not Applicable

[5] Safety, Health and Environmental

[6] In safety, health and environmental-related areas

[7] Where safety is at least 50%, preventative, professional level with breadth and depth of safety duties

[8] ASP, CIH, CMIOSH, CRSP, GSP, SISO, NEBOSH National or International Diploma in Occupational Health and Safety, Diploma in Industrial Safety from CLI/RLIs of the Government of India

[9] Where safety is at least 50%, preventative, professional level with breadth and depth of safety duties

[10] Must achieve the CSP within eligibility time period once CSP experience requirement is met

[11] A minimum of 35% of the job tasks must be related to management of safety related programs, processes, procedures, personnel, etc.)

[12] At least 35% of primary job duties involve safety and health

[13] At least 35% of primary job duties involve safety and health

[14] Related to the STS industry exam for which candidate is applying (work experience must be a minimum part time [18 hrs./week] to qualify)

[15] ASP, CDGP, CFPS CHMM, CHST, CIH, CMIOSH, CRSP, CSP, OHST, STS, or STSC

[16] Or by retaking the STS/STSC exam or earning the OHST, CHST, ASP or CSP

[17] With 2.8 of these points in attending a training, development or instructional technology class

About the CHST Exam

Shortly after the turn of the century there began appearing globally, persons practicing the art and science of safety work. These practitioners came from different academic backgrounds and had a multitude of work experience ranging from operations to engineering. They all had one common goal, promoting the safety and health of employees. Until the BCSP certification programs began, they also had no standard measure of qualification.

The Construction Health and Safety Technician® (CHST) is an accredited certification offered by the Board of Certified Safety Professionals (BCSP). The BSCP was chartered in 1969 to establish a method of measuring qualifications for the safety profession. The Board established qualification standards and began issuing certification shortly after being founding. Although chartered as an independent, separately-incorporated board, the BCSP has several sponsoring organizations which provide members to the BCSP Board of Directors. These sponsoring organizations are as follows:

- American Society of Safety Engineers (ASSE)

- American Industrial Hygiene Association (AIHA)

- National Safety Council (NSC)

- Institute of Industrial Engineers (IIE)

- Society of Fire Protection Engineers (SFPE)

- International System Safety Society (ISSS)

- National Fire Protection Association (NFPA)

- National Environmental Training Association (NESHTA)

CHST Qualifications

Candidates must meet experience and education/training requirements and pass a four-hour examination. Candidates for the CHST certification are typically employed as safety and health specialists on construction job sites, serving in either full-time or part-time positions. Typical individuals are responsible for safety and health on one or more significant construction projects or job sites. They may work for an owner, general contractor, subcontractor, or firm involved in construction or construction safety.

Candidates from various backgrounds can qualify for the CHST certification.

Candidates must meet the following requirements:
- Be of good moral character and have high ethical standards;
- Have experience in construction;
- Have health or safety training or education; and
- Pass the CHST examination.
- CHST must have a high school diploma or GED.
- Candidates need at least 3 years of construction experience with at least 35% safety duties.

Acceptable construction work experience includes:
- Work in a construction craft (e.g., carpenter, plumber, electrician, iron worker, millwright, painter, laborer, etc.).
- Work for a construction company as a manager, supervisor, or specialist that involves planning, organizing or executing construction projects that typically involve activities at or frequent visits to construction sites.
- Work as a designer or planner for construction projects.
- Work as a specialist for which the practice primarily involves construction.

Construction may involve activities related to the assembly, repair, and maintenance of buildings, earthworks, highways, bridges, structures, towers, tunnels, excavations, or other activities, such as quarrying and mining.

For more information about the qualifications, prerequisites and the application process for the CHST, please refer to the Complete Guide to the CHST. published by the BCSP.

Accredited Certification vs. Certificate Program

Accredited Certification	Certificate Program
Results from an assessment process	Results from an educational process
Typically requires some amount of professional experience	For novice and experienced professionals
Awarded by a third-party, standard-setting organization	Awarded by training and educational programs or institutions
Indicates master/competency as measured against a defensible set of standards, usually by application or exam	Indicates completion of a course or series of courses with a specific focus; is different than a degree granting program
Standards set through a defensible, industry-wide process (job analysis/role delineation) that results in an outline of required knowledge and skills	Course content set a variety of ways (faculty committee; dean; instructor; occasionally though defensible analysis of topic care)
Typically results in a designation to use after one's name; may result in a document to hang on the wall or keep in a wallet	Usually listed on a resume detailing education; may result in a document to hang on the wall
Has on-going requirements to maintain; individual must demonstrate knowledge of content; holder must demonstrate he/she continues to meet requirements	Is the end result; individual may or may not demonstrate knowledge of course content at the end of a set period in time

The BCSP's certifications are accredited by independent, third-party organizations that regularly evaluate certification requirements. Accreditation assures:

1. Governance
    - Nominations/elections
    - Peer participation
    - Public participation
2. Financial disclosure
    - Stability and financial condition
    - Budget details
3. Fairness to candidates
4. Examinations
    - Validity
    - Reliability
    - Passing scores
5. Recertification
6. Independence from preparation
7. Management systems

International Accreditation is provided by the American National Standards Institute (ANSI 17024/ISO)[18]. National Accreditation is achieved through both the National Commission for Certifying Agencies (NCCA)[19] and the Council of Engineering and Scientific Specialty Boards (CESB)[20].

---

[18] ASP, CSP
[19] ASP, CSP, OHST, CHST, STS
[20] CET

Benefits of Certification

The process of certification commands a considerable amount of effort. Many health & safety practitioners wonder if the advantages of certification justify all the effort. The primary advantage of certification is that it provides a credential. As the health and safety community gains a greater understanding of the CHST certification, the employment opportunities will increase for personnel holding certification. This has made the CHST a unique "stand-alone" certification that provides increased status for construction health and safety Practitioners. The CHST certification has maintained a high degree of credibility because of the affiliation with the BCSP.

The primary advantage of certification is that it provides a credential. The CHST indicates that a safety professional has achieved a standard level of qualification as judged by their professional peers. This level of qualification is important in establishing credibility within the ever-growing field of Occupational Health and Safety. Employment opportunities are much greater for personnel holding certification, the courts recognize the certification as a step toward authentication as an expert witness, and it is almost always required to do consultant work in the field of safety today. There are several reasons that should cause candidates to think about starting the process of obtaining certification *right now.*

- A growing trend by states to license safety professionals, much like physicians, engineers, architects, and other professionals. Some states have that authority under their duty to "protect the health, safety and welfare of the public."
- Substantial support to modify existing safety and health laws to acknowledge certified "safety specialists". Some projects require a certified professional to be on staff.
- Certified Safety and Health professionals obtain employment earlier and receive greater compensation than non-certified employees.
- As the requirements increase, the examinations may become even more dynamic, complex, difficult to pass and expensive, both in time and financial investments.

These and other recent developments add up to a future environment where a certification is going to be the desired/required credential. Being a CHST will become much more important, more lucrative, and more difficult to obtain. Like the other professional certification/registration examinations, the CHST exams should be taken as early in one's career as possible.

Overview of the CHST Certification Process

The following information concerning the requirements for certification may have changed after publication. It is strongly suggested candidates contact the BCSP for current information. For exact requirements, go to the BCSP web site at www.bcsp.org and review the CHST complete guide. There are common questions by potential candidates such as "What do I have to do to get the CHST?"

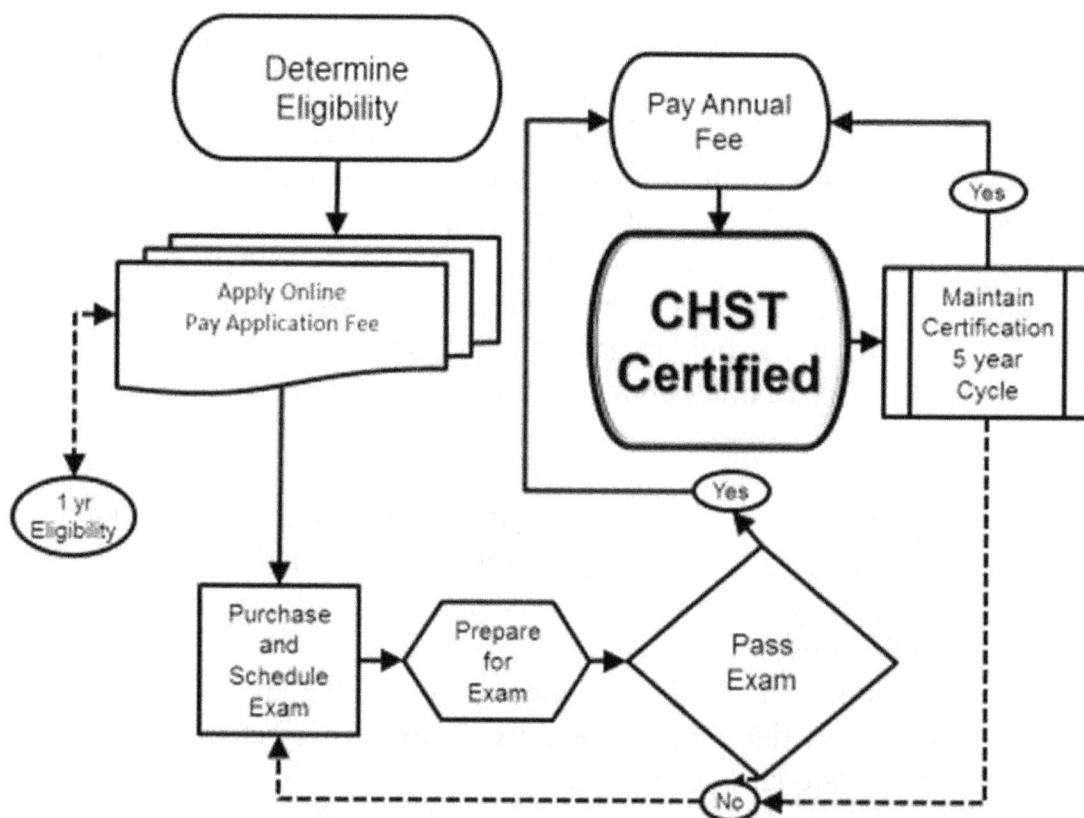

Applicants for CHST certification must be of high moral character and possess high ethical standards. They must document a history of three years of experience in occupational health or safety activities acceptable to the BCSP. Additionally, they must possess a high school diploma, or equivalent and pass a four-hour, 200 multiple choice question examination. To be considered, 35% of the applicant's time must have been spent in the field of occupational health or safety during the periods claimed for credit.

The entire process of certification generally takes from 3 to 6 months, allowing plenty of time to **PLAN** an individual study program. Costs associated with the certification process are as follows:

CHST Criteria	
Minimum Formal Education	High School diploma or GED
Training Prerequisite	N/A
Work Experience	At least 3 years of experience where safety is at least 35%, preventative, professional level with breadth and depth of safety duties
Application Fees	$140
Examination Fees	$300
Eligibility Extension Fees	$100
Renewal Fees	$120
Passing Scores	66.3%
Recertification (5-year cycle)	20 points

The above information is accurate as of this printing. For more current information, candidates should contact the Board at:

Board of Certified Safety Professionals
8645 Guion Road
Indianapolis, IN 64268
Phone (317) 593-4800
Fax (317) 593-4400
www.bcsp.org

Pearson VUE Testing Center Locations

For worldwide locations, look at the web site www.pearsonvue.com.
For all areas not listed, contact the BCSP for testing information.

The CHST Examination Blueprint

BCSP examination blueprints are based on surveys of what safety professionals do in practice. The CHST examination is required for candidates to demonstrate knowledge of professional safety practice at the CHST level. The top levels, called domains, represent the major functions performed by safety professionals at the CHST level. Each domain is divided among several topics listing knowledge and skill areas of that domain. Each domain heading is accompanied by a percentage label which represents the proportion of the actual CHST examination devoted to that domain effective in the 4th quarter 2018.

Domain 1: Hazard Identification and Control	57.1%
Domain 2: Emergency Preparedness and Fire Prevention	10.3%
Domain 3: Safety Program Development and Implementation	17.1%
Domain 4: Leadership, Communication and Training	15.5%

Domain one represents 57.1% of the exam, approximately 115 questions.
Domain two represents 10.3% of the exam, approximately 20 questions.
Domain three represents 17.1% of the exam, approximately 35 questions.
Domain four represents 15.5% of the exam, approximately 30 questions.

Of the 200-question exam, only 175 are scored, with 25 unscored experimental questions. The exam generates experimental questions that are not scored. These questions are measured by psychometric statistics to ensure validity and reliability before placed as a useable question in the exam database.

The CHST certification exam is designed to measure the broad spectrum of fundamental knowledge required in professional safety practice. Accordingly, many basic questions on the application of science, engineering and management fundamentals will be encountered. While some items test applied knowledge, the applications are basic; typically dealing with simple rather than complex problems, calculations and situations.

The computerized test consists of 200 questions covering four domains, and candidates are allowed four consecutive hours to complete all sections.

Domain 1: Hazard Identification and Control

Domain 1 *Hazard Identification and Control (includes Health Hazards)* • 57.1 %

Knowledge of:

1. Common hazards and controls associated with hot work (e.g., cutting, welding, grinding)
2. Common electrical hazards and controls
3. Common hazards and controls associated with excavations
4. Common hazards and controls associated with working at heights (e.g., ladders, scaffolding, aerial platforms)
5. Common hazards and controls associated with working in confined spaces
6. Common struck by hazards and associated controls
7. Common caught-in or caught-between hazards and associated controls
8. Common hazards and controls associated with hoisting and rigging
9. Common hazards and controls associated with crane operations
10. Common hazards and controls associated with material handling
11. Common hazards and controls associated with material storage
12. Common hazards and controls associated with housekeeping
13. Common hazards and controls associated with powder actuated tools
14. Common hazards and controls associated with hand and power tools
15. Common hazards and controls associated with asbestos exposure
16. Common hazards and controls associated with lead exposure
17. Common hazards and controls associated with noise exposure
18. Common hazards and controls associated with radiation exposure (ionizing and non-ionizing)
19. Common hazards and controls associated with silica exposure
20. Common hazards and controls associated with chemical exposure
21. Common hazards and controls associated with working in extreme temperatures
22. Common hazards and controls associated with vibration and impact exposures
23. The Globally Harmonized System of Classification and Labeling of Chemicals (GHS)
24. Basic safety through design (e.g., incorporating hierarchy of controls into design of building or systems)
25. Risks associated with multiple trades working simultaneously in work area (e.g., congested area, overlapping of workers)
26. Principles of ergonomics as applied to construction practices and material handling
27. Requirements, usage, and limitations of personal protective equipment
28. Basic testing and monitoring equipment (e.g., electrical, industrial hygiene, four gas meter) required for a situation

Skill to:

1. Apply the hierarchy of controls
2. Verify corrective actions were effective in eliminating or mitigating hazards
3. Recognize and address hazards over changing construction site conditions (e.g., excavations after weather events, changing site entrances)
4. Develop job/hazard safety analyses
5. Prioritize identified hazards based on level of risk (e.g., order of severity, probability, frequency)

Domain 2: Emergency Preparedness and Fire Prevention

Domain 2 *Emergency Preparedness and Fire Prevention • 10.3%*
Knowledge of:
1. Proper fire protection and prevention methods (e.g., appropriate class of fire extinguishers, inspection criteria)
2. Components of emergency action plans
3. Common elements of response plans for environmental hazards (e.g., releases or spills)
4. Emergency response system (e.g., incident command system, crisis management, emergency response equipment, media)
5. Potential first aid or medical needs (e.g., availability of first aid kit, AED, CPR supplies)
6. Universal precautions (e.g., bloodborne/airborne pathogens)
Skill to:
1. Plan for emergencies

Domain 3: Safety Program Development and Implementation

Domain 3 *Safety Program Development and Implementation • 17.1%*
Knowledge of:
1. Applicable health and safety standards and best practices (e.g., health, safety, construction, and environmental)
2. Common components of site-specific safety plans
3. Worksite assessment or audit processes
4. Roles, responsibilities, and lines of authority as they relate to safety management
5. Recommended equipment inspection records or logs
6. Basic risk management concepts (e.g., public safety, builder's risk and liabilities, general liability)
7. General/basic construction site conditions that could potentially impact safety
8. Data gathering techniques and procedures used in incident investigations
9. Techniques for determining the root cause of accidents or incidents
10. Post-incident/accident reporting and follow-up procedures
11. Documentation requirements of occupational injuries and illnesses
Skill to:
1. Identify which health and safety programs (e.g., fall protection, ladders, respiratory) are relevant to site-specific safety plan
2. Apply relevant standards to worksite conditions
3. Identify trends related to incidents and accidents
4. Evaluate construction means and methods and their impact on safety

Domain 4: Leadership, Communication, and Training

Domain 4 *Leadership, Communication, and Training* • 15.5%
Knowledge of:
1. Available training delivery methods and instructional materials (e.g., classroom, on-the-job training, online)
2. Appropriate human behavior motivation methods and techniques (e.g., behavior-based safety)
3. Communication strategies (e.g., methods to disseminate information)
4. When to consult with equipment manufacturers, suppliers, or subject matter experts
5. Information confidentiality requirements (e.g., trade secrets, personal medical, personally identifiable information)
6. BCSP Code of Ethics
Skill to:
1. Develop site-specific safety training requirements based on job tasks and work environment
2. Maintain all applicable documentation (e.g., training documents, injury logs)
3. Determine training requirements and delivery methods based on characteristics and needs of worksite personnel (e.g., skill level, education level, language proficiency)
4. Identify existing and foreseeable at-risk conditions and behaviors
5. Recognize situations or behaviors that present imminent danger
6. Coach personnel to correct unsafe behaviors
7. Access relevant current information (e.g., standards, codes, safety-related information)
8. Apply the BCSP Code of Ethics

Taking the Computer Based Exam

One major goal of the BCSP is to offer certification examinations with a high degree of validity and reliability to promote a fair assessment of a candidate's competency as a safety and health practitioner.

Testing on computer is done via Pearson VUE (www.pearsonvue.com) Examinations can be taken every business day at many locations throughout the world. Many locations also have evening and Saturday hours.

Candidates must complete an application and return it, supporting information and application fee ($140) to the Board of Certified Safety Professionals (BCSP). Once a candidate has been approved and has paid the examination fee ($300), the Board will mail an examination authorization letter. Once the application is approved, candidates have one year to arrange for an actual examination date. Arrangements are made directly with Pearson VUE via on-line or via the national toll-free number **888.269.2219**. Some Pearson VUE Testing Centers are busier than others, so schedule early if possible.

At the Pearson VUE centers, a candidate signs in, presents identifications and is seated at a computer workstation. The center provides laminated graph paper and a marker. There is a short orientation and practice program to acquaint candidates with the examination procedure. During actual testing a small clock in the monitor screen corner keeps track of the remaining time.

ABSOLUTELY NO NOTES OR REFERENCE MATERIALS ARE ALLOWED! Laminated graphing paper and writing utensils will be provided. After finishing the computerized examination, a pass-fail grade will be given. A detailed score report will be mailed later from the BCSP.

For worldwide locations, look at the web site www.pearsonvue.com.

Frequently Asked Questions about the Computer Exam

NOTE: Remember the best and most current source of information on procedures and policies for the computer test is directly from the BCSP at (317) 593-4800 and www.bcsp.org.

Question   How do the questions appear on the computer screen? How do I make answer selections? Can I back up or mark questions so that I can come back to them? Do I need to be a computer whiz to take this test?

Answer   Examination questions appear one at a time and look very similar to the questions in the workbook. With a mouse or keys, the candidate selects the preferred answer and moves on to the next question. Questions may be marked for further review or skipped and revisited later. After the last question, a list appears and shows item numbers, answers selected, and questions marked or skipped. Since the computer test is very "friendly" candidates do not have to be computer literate to take this exam.

Question   Can you bring food or drinks into the exam room?

Answer   No. All candidates are given a small locker for personal belongings, including snacks, purses, watches, etc. Access to this locker may or may not be allowed depending upon the testing center.

Question   What can I take into the exam room?

Answer   ID cards are permitted. Everything else must go into personal lockers.

Question   What is furnished in the exam cubicle?

Answer   One laminated sheet of paper, one marker and the computer monitor, keyboard and mouse.

Question   What is the workstation/cubicle like?

Answer   It is generally very nice, although this may vary with different Pearson VUE Centers. Cubicles are large, with a desktop about 3'x 4', excellent lighting, in a very quiet setting, with comfortable, padded adjustable chairs. The keyboard and mouse take up all space in front of the monitor, so calculations must be done off to the side.

Question   Are there any children in the exam room?

Answer   No. The room is for adult testing only. All children activities are in separate areas of the Pearson VUE Center.

Question   How many other people are in the room?

Answer   There are multiple workstations in the exam room. The number of people varies with time and day. The proctor has a view of the entire room via glass window and corner mirrors on the ceiling. Testing is also taped by video and audio monitoring.

Question   Can I take breaks?

Answer   Yes, as many and as often as necessary. However, the clock keeps running and signing out is required each time, along with a finger print check.

Question   Do I need ID's?

Answer   One ID with photo and signature is mandatory. Photograph and a finger print are done during sign-in.

Question   Do I need my Authorization letter with Candidate ID Number?

Answer   This letter is usually not required, but it is advised to take it just in case. The ID number is always needed when scheduling examination appointments.

Question   Can I schedule the exam any time?

Answer   No. Certain times are designated for professional exams. Book testing slot several weeks in advance to secure the desired time and day.

Question   Is there enough time to finish the exam?

Answer   This is very subjective. Most candidates have found there was plenty of time to finish testing and have adequate review time, but other people did not finish in the allotted time. The time per question (1.5 minutes) is the same as the written exam and the authors found the computer not to be a factor in this area.

Question   Are there graphs to interpret? How are clear are the graphics?

Answer   Yes, there are a limited number of graphs to read. They are a little harder to read on the screen, but not significantly. Graphics are quite acceptable.

Question   Are the math formulas provided?

Answer   If a problem required a formula(s), then they should be provided in the question.

The computer exam is a positive, convenient way to take the exam. The Pearson VUE people were friendly and helpful. The cubicles are quiet and well-lit and the chairs are relatively comfortable. There is adequate table space and the computer was user friendly and non-threatening.

Conditions may vary considerably between testing locations. Please contact authors at 417-724-8348 or Email info@spansafetyworkshops.com. Feedback is greatly appreciated.

A listing of Pearson VUE center locations is available through the Pearson VUE website. More complete information can be obtained by calling or faxing the Board of Certified Safety Professionals. **Good Luck on the exam!**

Applied Study & Testing Techniques

The examination blueprint outlines how the items on an examination are distributed across domains and tasks/topics. Some keys to success include:

1. Analyzing knowledge gaps and identify strengths and weaknesses
2. Designing a solid examination study plan
3. Developing test-taking strategies

Converting your subject strengths and weaknesses into a study plan is likely to increase your overall examination score. Scoring well in one subject area can compensate for a weaker score in another subject area. However, there may not be enough items in your strong areas to achieve a passing score.
Note that knowledge and understanding are essential in passing the examination. Relying only on simulated examination items is not the best way to increase knowledge and understanding. Use simulated items to provide insight into the areas in which you should engage in additional study.

Knowing how to take the examination will help improve your score. The examination uses multiple-choice items with only one correct answer and three incorrect answers. Remember, the goal is to get as many items correct as possible. There is no penalty for selecting an incorrect answer. However, only correct answers count toward reaching the passing score.

- Read the items carefully.
    - Psychometricians design multiple choice questions so that all the possible answer choices are plausible. Use deductive and inductive reasoning to eliminate detractor answer choices.
- Understand the problem.
    - Consider the context
    - What is given? What is wanted?
- Use examination time wisely.
    - Conduct multiple passes solving the "easy" problems first and saving the challenging problems for the end.
- Complete all items.
    - Blank answers are scored as wrong answers.

While studying resources, identify main thoughts or themes in the literature review. Draw on your experience and on professional and study references and rewrite important ideas in your own words. This helps you remember the concepts in context. Additional references are listed later in the workbook.

In establishing a good study regiment, it is important to find a place conducive to studying. A good study area should meet the following criteria:

- The study place should be chosen exclusively for studying. Avoid using a garage, workshop, family room or other area that represents recreation or other distractions. Find a location that represents a study island, where study is the **only** activity.
- Selected study area should have good lighting, ventilation, be temperature controlled, comfortable and quiet.
- A large table or desk to spread necessary readily available study and reference materials is a must. The purpose is to dedicate a comfortable, personal space with minimal interruptions.

Securing a good place to study should eliminate as many external distractions as possible. Also, candidates should consider how to minimize internal distractions. Total elimination of external distractions is often possible; however, total elimination of internal distractions is nearly impossible and can only be minimized through focused thought.

Helpful hints for focusing the mind for studying include the following:

1. Set realistic time limits, determining what to study and keeping with a schedule. Studying a subject too long at one time can lead to daydreaming which reduces study effectiveness.

2. Personal factors can be distracters and result in additional frustration. All efforts should be attempted in avoiding personal issues. Rescheduling the CHST test date may be a consideration if serious personal problems exist.

3. Minimize dealing with outside details. Having too many obligations and/or responsibilities enables "brain creep". Consider keeping a notebook in the study area and jotting down appointments and details of projects as these brainstorms appear. It's impossible to totally prevent these details from surfacing, but by documenting them, it may free the mind to resume studies.

4. Being physically and mentally prepared to study is beneficial. Much of the following suggestions are common sense, but probably deserve repeating.

   o Eat a well-balanced diet. Increase protein intake; a proper level of blood sugar enhances studying effectiveness.
   o Get plenty of sleep. Establish and maintain a regular work/rest cycle.
   o Exercise is beneficial for more than just an exam preparation. Consider choosing a form of exercise that provides enjoyment and relaxation.
   o Avoid mental fatigue. Allocate down time for breaks. The average supervisor should study for the CHST exam for two to four weeks. DO NOT attempt to cram overnight.

The Question/Answer Study Method

The Volume I and II workbooks apply a Question & Answer format that allows candidates to concentrate on knowledge gaps and avoid over studying material in areas where the candidate already possess enough knowledge to pass the exam.

The authors have researched the blueprint areas of interest, developing targeted learning outcomes. This allows candidates to determine if their current level knowledge is adequate, or if a more in-depth understanding is required.

Fundamental to this technique is a good core of questions. The technique is intended to be useful to practitioners who have mastered the skills and tasks necessary to perform in the safety and health arena.

Most adult learners enjoy the process of learning. The difference lies in the ability to retain what is important to the accomplishment of a goal and reject what is not important. Embrace the aspect of professional development while preparing for the CHST examination.

When utilizing this workbook properly, the authors believe candidates can master those areas necessary to achieve the goal of passing the CHST examination with minimum effort on research and actual study. The technique also has some very beneficial side effects. Candidates will also find that the learning process will enhance skill sets in becoming an improved and more proficient safety and health practitioner.

However, the process assumes candidates have the discipline to do the research and study the material where deficiencies may exist. Attempting to study using only the material presented in this workbook, becomes a risk for not being adequately prepared for the examination.

The steps to using the Q & A method:

1. Dead reckoning: use existing knowledge, experience, and test taking strategies, answer the question through logic and reasoning.

2. Process check: review the results of each practice session, and then study the explanation.

3. Validate knowledge: was this a known or an unknown concept? Is the answer achieved with current knowledge base or by an educated guess or dumb luck?

Note: This is a critical step in the Q&A learning process and determines if one can proceed or needs to gain more knowledge on the subject. Additionally, is the knowledge base on this subject broad enough to answer questions of similar difficulty on the subject? *"True genius is an uncluttered mind armed with only relevant knowledge"(John R. Monteith).*

4. Filter: either move on or take notes. When comfortable with knowledge on the subject move on to the next question. However, if the current level of knowledge on the subject or other aspects of the subject feels inadequate, then research and take additional notes about the information. Write in the workbook margins right next to the question.

5. Enhance deficiencies: Research and study deficient knowledge areas. After completing a set of questions and writing notes on information to study, a knowledge deficiency study plan can be developed. Then research and study the material necessary to enhance the required knowledge. The authors advise focusing on notes in the workbook and staying on subject. It is very easy to wander onto some other interesting subject and lose sight of the desired learning outcome. Keep the goal in mind to pass the test the first time!

Applied Logic: Socratic Method

Consider this representative question, answer and explanation to illustrate and explain the learning process.

Question:

Which is the most correct statement about the function of an electrical Ground Fault Circuit Interrupter (GFCI)?

A.) It is a slow acting device.
B.) It interrupts the electric power within 1/40th of a second.
C.) It will detect line-to-line faults.
D.) It is not designed for personnel protection.

YOUR NAME | Question: 01 of 200
CHST Exam version | Time remaining: 320 min

Which is the most correct statement about the function of an electrical Ground Fault Circuit Interrupter (GFCI)?

O A.) It is a slow acting device.
B.) It interrupts the electric power within 1/40th of a second.
O C.) It will detect line-to-line faults.
O D.) It is not designed for personnel protection.

FURTHER REVIEW | PREVIOUS | NEXT

Answer:

The most correct answer is B.

Explanation: A **GFCI** is specifically designed to **protect people** against electric shock from an electrical system, and it monitors the imbalance of current between the ungrounded (hot) and grounded (neutral) conductor of a given circuit. *These devices will operate on a circuit that does not have an equipment-grounding conductor.* Except for small amounts of leak-age, the current returning to the power supply in a typical 2-wire circuit will be equal to the current leaving the power supply. If the difference between the current leaving and returning through the current transformer of the GFCI (leakage) exceeds **5 mA**, the solid-state circuitry opens the switching contacts and de-energizes the circuit. Whenever the amount *going* differs from the amount *returning* by a set trip level the GFCI interrupts the electric power within **1/40th** of a second.

How much will candidates need to know about the subject of GFCIs? If electrical work represents a strong area, a candidate probably has significant knowledge about the GFCI and is comfortable with this question and the general subject. Another possibility is that one is basically knowledgeable on the subject, but could use some more focused descriptors. Another scenario may be that a candidate knows very little about GFCIs, requiring more focus on concept details and application techniques. How far into the topic does a student need to explore? The level of detail in the example question may serve as a representative indicator. Beyond the basics, another key indicator is the repetition of the workbook question. Content frequently appearing with only minor changes in question format indicates that the subject matter is important, and authors anticipate the actual exam will have several questions dealing with that subject.

The Q & A method of studying is a proven method. The basic outline is delivered with questions and students can then determine individual levels of subject knowledge. When additional knowledge is required, they can conduct more research and study to develop the required knowledge or skill. This learning technique has proven to be successful for many different levels of adult learners because **the individual** determines what material to study.

Example Computer Graphic User Interface

Compute the total power consumed for this simple parallel circuit.

O A.) 13.8 W

B.) 57 W

O C.) 414 W

O D.) 571 W

$$\frac{1}{R_{PARALLEL}} = \frac{1}{R_1} + \frac{1}{R_2} + \cdots + \frac{1}{R_N}$$

$$E = IR \qquad P = EI$$

$10\,\Omega \qquad 10\,\Omega \qquad 10\,\Omega$

Formulas will be inserted into the question when needed

13.8 volts

FURTHER REVIEW   PREVIOUS   NEXT

The purpose of the jockey pump is to maintain the fire sprinkler system _____ .

O A.) Total pressure.

B.) Static pressure

O C.) Residual pressure

O D.) Maximum pressure

The Jockey pump is designed prevent false starts of the fire pump and to start before the main fire pump and return the fire protection system to its minimum static pressure.

NFPA 20 Stationary Pumps

Pump: 1000-gpm, 100-psi pump with churn pressure of 115 psi.
Fire Pump start 150 psi
Fire pump stop 165 psi

Fire pump controller

Optional City Main Bypass

Minimum 5 ft (1.5 m)

Fire Alarm Check Valve

Water supply

Fire pump

Fire protection system

Supply:
50 psi min static.
60 psi max static.

Jockey pump

Minimum 5 ft (1.5 m)

Jockey pump:
start 155 psi
stop 165 psi

Jockey pump controller

FURTHER REVIEW   PREVIOUS   NEXT   EXHIBIT   REVIEW

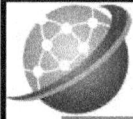

CHST Exam Math and Science

The Math and Science part of the Volume I workbook provides a foundation review. It is designed to allow you to become familiar with performing calculations like the ones encountered on the CHST examination. Several additional representative math questions may be found in the Volume II workbook.

Candidates will be provided an on-screen calculator during their exam. The on-screen calculator will emulate the TI-30XS scientific calculator. Test centers do not provide physical calculators or allow candidates to bring in their own. Please visit the BCSP website for the current calculator policy.

CHST Math Questions Quiz 1

1). For the excavation shown, what is the slope of side "C"?
$$a^2 + b^2 = c^2$$

A) ¼:1
B) ½:1
C) 1:1
D) 1 ½: 1

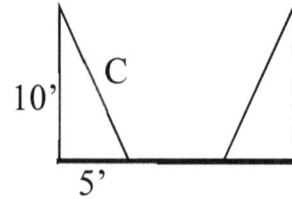

2). How much does a 55-gallon drum of acid weigh the acid is 2.1? Note: Water weighs 8.34 pounds per gallon?

A) 460
B) 1700
C) 802
D) 965

3). A standpipe 95 feet high, radius of 3 inches, filled with water creates _____ psi?

A) 41 psi
B) 38 psi
C) 30.5 psi
D) 10 psi

4). A 1200-pound load is lifted with a 2 leg sling whose legs are at a 30 degree angle with the load. The stress on each leg of the sling is:

$$\sin A = \frac{a}{c} \quad \cos A = \frac{b}{c} \quad \text{Tan } A = \frac{a}{b}$$

A) 600 lbs
B) 1200 lbs
C) 2400 lbs
D) 3600 lbs

5). A train carrying industrial chemicals is traveling at 120 mph. The engineer's reaction time is 0.9 seconds. How many feet will the locomotive travel before the engineer recognizes an emergency and applies the brakes?
   A) 265 feet.
   B) 260 feet.
   C) 160 feet.
   D) 165 feet.

6). Management has proposed to install a new manufacturing unit on the second floor of one of the buildings. The unit is 12 feet by 12 feet square and weighs 18,000 pounds total. When you are doing you initial evaluation of the proposal, you find engineering drawings that state "the maximum floor loading for the proposed location is 150 PSF. Can the unit be installed safely?
   A) No, the loading is over maximum by 10 PSF.
   B) No, the loading is over maximum by 25 PSF.
   C) Yes, the loading is under maximum by 10 PSF.
   D) Yes, the loading is under maximum by 25 PSF.

7). Compute the TWA concentration from the following measurement data: 0700-1000 hrs. @ 100 ppm---1000-1200 hrs. @ 200 ppm---1300-1400 hrs. @ 0 ppm and 1400-1600 hrs. @ 100 ppm.

$$ppm = \frac{(C_1 \times T_1) + (C_2 \times T_2) + (C_3 \times T_3) + (C_4 \times T_4)}{T_1 + T_2 + T_3 + T_4}$$

   A) 100 ppm
   B) 133.3 ppm
   C) 112.5 ppm
   D) 122 ppm

8). A reading of 2.5 percent hydrogen in air is equal to how many parts per million (ppm)?
   A) 43,250 ppm
   B) 2000 ppm
   C) 25,000 ppm
   D) 250,000 ppm

9). The atmospheric concentration of benzene is 9.2 ppm, and the MW of benzene is 78. What is the concentration in mg/m^3?

A) 29.3 mg/m^3
B) 19.2 mg/m^3
C) 49.2 mg/m^3
D) 69.2 mg/m^3

$$ppm = \frac{mg/m^3 \times 24.45}{MW}$$

10). Assuming complete evaporation and no air change, does the concentration created by the following conditions exceed the LEL? A leak in a pressurized piping system sprays 5 gallons of Ethyl alcohol in a room that is 15 feet by 15 feet by 8 feet. The molecular weight of Ethyl alcohol is 46 and the SG is 0.6. LEL is 3.3%.

A) Yes, more than 3 times the LEL
B) No, 50% of the LEL
C) No, 25% of the LEL
D) Yes, 10% over LEL

$$ppm = \frac{mg/m^3 \times 24.45}{MW}$$

11). If the measured noise level of an industrial motor vehicle is 77 dBA at a distance of 60 feet, what is the sound pressure level at 15 feet?

$$dB_1 = dB_0 + 20\log_{10}\left(\frac{d_0}{d_1}\right)$$

A) 80 dB
B) 89 dB
C) 98 dB
D) 85 dB

12). What is the combined Sound Pressure Level from two identical machines located adjacent to each other, if each machine is producing 85 dBA? What would the combined SPL be if there were four machines, 7 machines and 11 machines?

A) 88, 91, 93.5, & 95.4 dBA
B) 91, 97, 101, & 105.5 dBA
C) 88, 91, 95, & 97 dBA
D) 88, 91, 93, & 96 dBA

$$SPL_T = SPL_I + 10\log n$$

13). If a worker's noise exposure is 165% after 8 hours of noise exposure, what would be the TWA for the 8-hour period?

A) 165 dB
B) 93.6 dB
C) 93.25 dB
D) 126.83 dB

$$TWA = 90 + 16.61 \times LOG \left[\frac{D\%}{100} \right]$$

14). Based on the allowable limits in the table below if the noise in a work area was 95 dBA for 3 hrs, 90 dBA for 5 hrs and 85 dBA for 2 hrs, is the allowable limit exceeded?

PERMISSIBLE NOISE EXPOSURES					
Hrs	dBA	Hrs	dBA	Hrs	dBA
8	90	3	97	1	105
6	92	2	100	0.5	110
4	95	1.5	102	0.25	115

A) Yes, by more than 40%
B) No, less than 30 % exposure.
C) No, less than 50% exposure.
D) Yes, by more than 50%.

15). Using the following formula, evaluate the effectiveness of the hearing protection provided to a employee who is using an ear plug assigned a NRR of 29 combined with muffs (NRR = 25) when exposed to an 8 hour TWA of 110 dBA. Note: When two noise reduction devices are used, calculate the attenuation based on the most effective and add 5 for the second.

$$A_f = \frac{NRR - 7}{2}$$

A) Protected TWA = 99
B) Protected TWA = 94
C) Protected TWA = 110
D) Protected TWA = 84

16). A radioisotope has a half-life of 1 year. How many years will it take to reduce the initial activity to less than 10%?

- A) 1 year.
- B) 2 years.
- C) 3 years.
- D) 4 years.

CHST Math Answers Quiz 1

1)   Answer B:

Slope = Run over Rise

Slope – 5/10 or ½:1

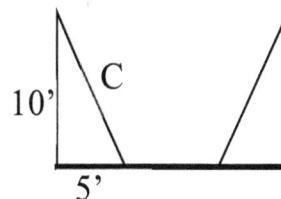

2)   Answer D:

Specific gravity (SG) is the ratio of a substance compared to an equal volume of water. In this case one gallon of acid weighs 2.1 times the weight of water. The formula then becomes # of gallons $\times 8.34 \times$ SG.

$55 \times 8.34 \times 2.1 = 963.3$ lbs

3)   Answer A is correct:

The constant for water pressure is 0.433 psi per foot of elevation.

$0.433 \times 95 = 41.135$.
Water has a weight density of 62.4 lbs/ft^3
$62.4 \div (12 \times 12) = 0.433$ psi/ft of elevation.

4) Answer B:

Step 1.   Draw right triangle and label.

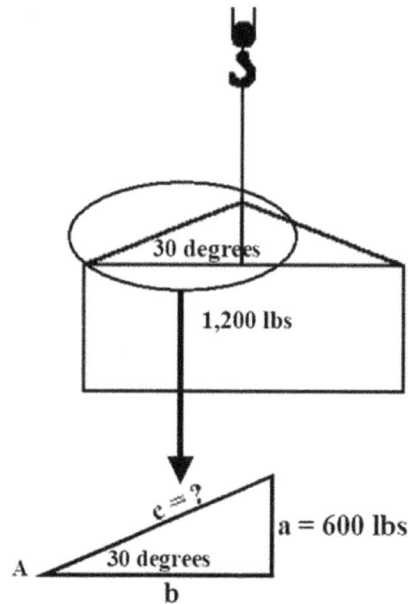

Note: There are two slings, so you could draw either "right triangle". We chose the left by convention. Solution for the right side would yield the same answer. Additionally, since there are two slings the total weight divides by two.

Step 2.   Apply formula, rearrange and solve for the unknown.

HINT: Double divided SLINGS are SIN full. Divide the load by two (number of sling legs) and then divide again by the SIN of the angle.

$$\sin A = \frac{a}{c}$$

$$1200 \div 2 \div \sin 30 = 1,200 \text{ lbs}$$

$$c = \frac{a}{\sin A}$$

$$c = \frac{600}{\sin 30}$$

$$c = 1200 \text{lbs}$$

5) Answer C:

$$\text{Distance} = \text{Speed times Time.}$$

$$D = \frac{(120 \times 5280)}{(60 \times 60)} \times 0.9 \text{ seconds}$$

$$D = 158.2 \text{ feet}$$

HINT: $5280 \div 3600 = 1.47$ (a constant that is often used in these type of problems) 1.47 times MPH = feet per second
$120 \times 1.47 \times 0.9 = 158.8$ feet

6) Answer D:

$$\text{Total ft}^2 \text{ of Unit} = 12 \text{ ft} \times 12 \text{ ft} = 144 \text{ ft}^2$$

$$\text{PSF for Unit} = \frac{18000 \text{ lbs}}{144 \text{ ft}^2} = 125 \text{ PSF}$$

Therefore, the PSF of the unit is 25 PSF under the maximum of 150 PSF.

7) Answer C:

$$\text{ppm} = \frac{(C_1 \times T_1) + (C_2 \times T_2) + (C_3 \times T_3) + (C_4 \times T_4)}{T_1 + T_2 + T_3 + T_4}$$

$$\frac{300 + 400 + 0 + 200}{3 + 2 + 1 + 2} = \frac{900}{8} = 112.5$$

8) Answer C:

$$2.5\% = 0.025$$
$$0.025 \text{ times } 1,000,000 = 25,000$$

9) Answer A:

$$ppm = \frac{mg/m^3 \times 24.45}{MW}$$

ppm = parts per million in concentration
mg/m^3 = milligrams/cubic meter
MW = Molecular weight of the substance

$$ppm = \frac{mg/m^3 \times 24.45}{MW}$$

$$mg/m^3 = \frac{MW \times ppm}{24.45}$$

$$mg/m^3 = \frac{78 \times 9.2}{24.45} = 29.3 \, mg/m^3$$

10) Answer A:

Step 1: Determine Volume in m^3

$$\frac{15 \, ft}{1} \times \frac{.305 \, m}{1 \, ft} = 4.6 \, m$$

$$\frac{8 \, ft}{1} \times \frac{.305 \, m}{1 \, ft} = 2.44 \, m$$

$$4.6 \times 4.6 \times 2.44 = 51.6 \, m^3$$

Step 2:   Determine weight

$$\frac{5 \text{ gal}}{1} \times \frac{8.34 \text{ lbs}}{\text{gal}} \times 0.6 = 25 \text{ lbs}$$

Step 3:   Convert- lbs to mg

$$\frac{25 \text{ lb}}{1} \times \frac{.4545 \text{ kg}}{1 \text{ lb}} \times \frac{1000 \text{g}}{1 \text{ kg}} \times \frac{1000 \text{ mg}}{1 \text{ g}}$$

$$= 11,362,500$$

$$= 1.14 \times 10^{7} \text{ mg}$$

Step 4:   Compute-ppm

$$\text{ppm} = \frac{\text{mg/m}^{3} \times 24.45}{\text{MW}}$$

$$\text{ppm} = \frac{(1.14 \times 10^{7}/51.6) \times 24.45}{46}$$

$$\text{ppm} = 117,043$$

Step 5: Convert to %

$$\left(\frac{117,043}{1,000,000} \right) \times 100 = 11.7\%$$

Alternate Solution

Step 1:   Determine- Volume

$$15 \times 15 \times 8 = 1800 \text{ ft}^{3}$$

Step 2:   Determine-
weight

$$\frac{5\text{ gal}}{1} \times \frac{8.345\text{ lbs}}{\text{gal}} \times 0.6 = 25\text{ lbs}$$

Step 3:   Determine the volume occupied by the Ethyl alcohol

$$\frac{46\text{ lbs}}{392\text{ ft}^3} = \frac{25\text{ lbs}}{X}$$

$$X = \frac{25 \times 392}{46}$$

$$X = 213\text{ ft}^3$$

Step 4:   Determine concentration of Ethyl alcohol in the 1800 ft^3 room.

$$\frac{213\text{ ft}^3}{1800\text{ ft}^3} \times 100 = 11.8\%$$

11)   Answer B:

As the distance from the source doubles the noise decreases 6 dB. Since the distance from the source has halved twice, the net change is 12 dB. $77 + 12 = 89$ dBA. At 7.5 ft the level is $89 + 6 = 95$ dBA and at 3.75 feet the noise level is $95 + 6 = 101$ dBA and so on.

$$dB_0 = 77\text{ dB}$$
$$dB_1 = ?$$
$$d_0 = 60\text{ft}$$
$$d_1 = 15\text{ft}$$

$$dB_1 = 77 + 20\log_{10}\left(\frac{60}{15}\right)$$

$$dB_1 = 77 + 20\log_{10}(4)$$

$$dB_1 = 77 + 12.04 = 89\text{ dB}$$

12) Answer A:

The simplified formula for calculation of equal Sound Pressure Levels is:

Two Machines

$$SPL_T = SPL_I + 10 \log n$$

$$SPL_T = 85 + 10 \times \log 2$$

$$SPL_T = 85 + 3.01 = 88.01 \, dB$$

Four Machines

$$SPL_T = SPL_I + 10 \log n$$

$$SPL_T = 85 + 10 \times \log 4$$

$$SPL_T = 85 + 6.02 = 91.02 \, dB$$

Seven Machines

$$SPL_T = SPL_I + 10 \log n$$

$$SPL_T = 85 + 10 \times \log 7$$

$$SPL_T = 85 + 8.45 = 93.45 \, dB$$

Eleven Machines

$$SPL_T = SPL_I + 10 \log n$$

$$SPL_T = 85 + 10 \times \log 11$$

$$SPL_T = 85 + 10.41 = 95.41 \, dB$$

13) Answer B:

Compute TWA

$$TWA = 90 + 16.61 \times LOG \left[\frac{D\%}{100} \right]$$

$$TWA = 90 + 16.61 \times LOG \left[\frac{165}{100} \right]$$

$$TWA = 90 + 16.61 \times 0.2175 = 93.6$$

14) Answer A:

$$\frac{C_1}{T_1} + \frac{C_2}{T_2} + \frac{C_3}{T_3} = exposure$$

$$\frac{3}{4} + \frac{5}{8} + \frac{2}{no\ limit} = 1.375\ is > 1 \rightarrow exposure\ not\ allowed$$

15) Answer B:

$$A_f = \frac{NRR\ -\ 7}{2} + 5$$

$$A_f = \frac{29\ -\ 7}{2} + 5$$

$$A_f = 11 + 5$$

$$A_f = 16$$

$$Protected\ TWA = TWA_8 - A_f$$

$$Protected\ TWA = 110 - 16$$

$$Protected\ TWA = 94\ dBA$$

When trying to evaluate the impact of high noise levels on the human ear it is very difficult to determine the effectiveness of hearing protectors. Hearing protectors are evaluated under laboratory conditions specified by ANSI Z 24.22 and ANSI S 3.19. However, in field conditions the Noise Reduction Rating (NRR) given hearing protectors often is provided a safety factor of 2 or reduced by 50%. This is necessary because field conditions never equal laboratory conditions. Additionally, when two noise reduction devices are properly worn and additional 5 dB (doubling) of protection is provided. After the field attenuation is calculated it is subtracted from the 8 hour TWA value to obtain the protected TWA (sound level reaching the cochlea). If the variations in noise level involve maxima at intervals of 1 second or less, it is to be considered continuous.

TABLE G-16 - PERMISSIBLE NOISE EXPOSURES (1)

Duration per day, hours	Sound level dBA slow response
8	90

Exposure to impulsive or impact noise should not exceed 140 dB peak sound pressure level.

Employers shall ensure that hearing protectors are worn: By an employee who is required by paragraph (b)(1) of this section to wear personal protective equipment; and By any employee who is exposed to an 8-hour time-weighted average of 85 decibels or greater, and who: Has not yet had a baseline audiogram established pursuant to paragraph (g)(5)(ii); or Has experienced a **standard threshold shift**. For employees who have experienced a significant threshold shift, hearing protector attenuation must be sufficient to reduce employee exposure to a TWA of 85 dB.

Employees shall be given the opportunity to select their hearing protectors from a variety of suitable hearing protectors provided by the employer.

16) Answer D:

The activity after three years will be 12.5% of the initial activity. After 4 years the activity will be 6.25% of the initial activity.

$$100\% \quad 1^{st} \text{ yr} \quad = 50\%$$
$$50\% \quad 2^{nd} \text{ yr} \quad = 25\%$$
$$25\% \quad 3^{rd} \text{ yr} \quad = 12.5\%$$
$$12.5\% \quad 4^{th} \text{ yr} \quad = 6.25\%$$

CHST Math Questions Quiz 2

1) The mean plus or minus one standard deviation estimates what percentage of the distribution in a *normal* distribution?

   A) 95 %
   B) 99 %
   C) 68 %
   D) 50 %

2) In the following set of numbers, what is the median value?

   8, 8, 10, 12, 13, 15, 19

   A) 12
   B) 8
   C) 12.14
   D) 11

3) To select a system from among three potential safety design candidates, a Safety & Health consultant must recognize system failure will result in a loss, regardless of choice. An elementary design for each system showing probability of failure is shown below using standard "fault tree" symbols. Which system has the lowest overall failure probability?

   A) System A has lower probability and offers redundancy.
   B) System B has lower probability but has two potential single point failures.
   C) System C is the simplest and has lowest probability.
   D) The probability is the same for all three systems.

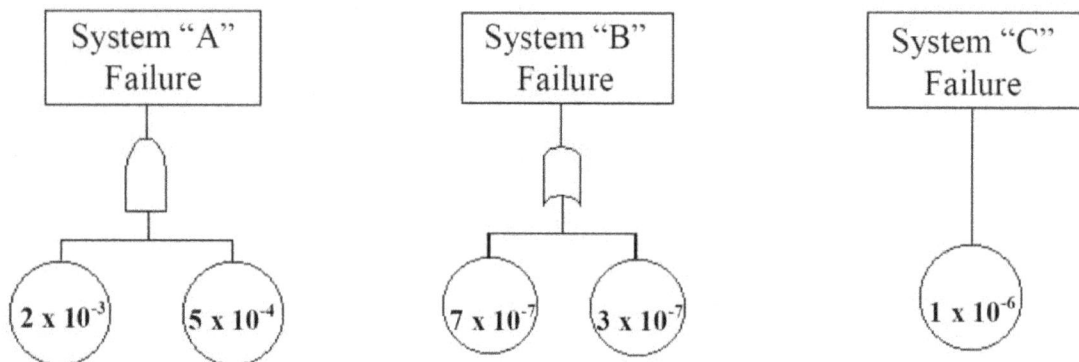

System "A" Failure	System "B" Failure	System "C" Failure
2×10^{-3} 5×10^{-4}	7×10^{-7} 3×10^{-7}	1×10^{-6}

4) Your Safety Committee is made up of 10 men and two women. What is the probability if you make a random selection of two individuals, that both individuals will be female?
   A) 0.007
   B) 0.028
   C) 0.015
   D) 0.167

5) Your plant has had 50 serious vehicle accidents in the past 10 years, three involving forklifts. What is the probability that the next serious accident will involve a forklift?
   A) 10%
   B) 5.0%
   C) 9.0%
   D) 6.0%

6) What is the vehicle accident rate of an operation experiencing 25 accidents while traveling 2,000,000 miles?
   A) 25 accidents per million miles
   B) 12.5 accidents per million miles
   C) 15 accidents per million miles
   D) 50 accidents per million miles

7) A company decides to reflect the worker's compensation losses against the profit function and to determine how many units must be sold to offset these costs. The profit margin of 2.5% on each unit sold and the worker's compensation for the last year were $90,000. What is the volume of sales needed to offset the worker's compensation losses?
   A) $600,000
   B) $3,000,000
   C) $3,600,000
   D) $30,000,000

8) ABC Manufacturing has a machine that has contributed to 14 employees being injured in the last 4 years. A retrofit has been proposed that will eliminate the hazard and its total cost is $30,000. The total direct cost of the employee injuries was $12,250. Without considering any indirect costs or the value of money, how many months will it take for the retrofit to pay for itself?

   A) 12
   B) 118
   C) 179
   D) 2143

9) Calculate the incidence rate for a company if the recordable accidents are 40 and the total hours are 1,500,000:

   A) 5.3
   B) 8.7
   C) 10.2
   D) 11.5

10) If a job site operation results in some $45,000 loss every three years, what is the expected loss over a period of 12 years?

   A) $180,000
   B) $270,000
   C) $250,000
   D) $360,000

11) If a Job site operation results in some $90,000 loss every three years, what is the expected loss over a period of 12 years?

   A) $180,000
   B) $270,000
   C) $250,000
   D) $360,000

CHST Math Answers Quiz 2

1)   Answer C:

The mean plus or minus one standard deviation will estimate the point at which 68% of the observations will fall.

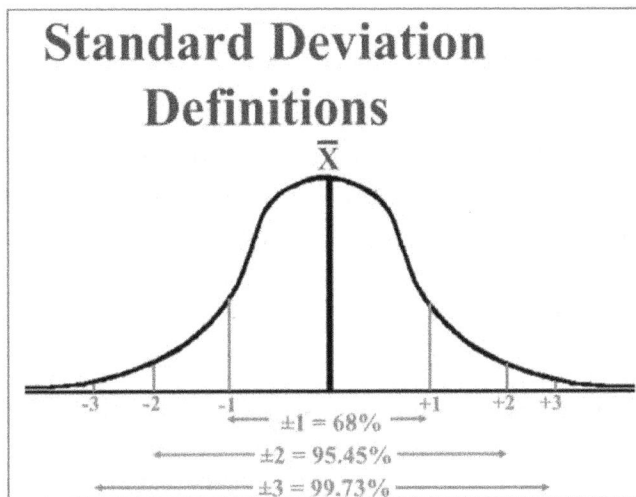

Standard Deviation Definitions

$\bar{X}$

-3   -2   -1   +1   +2   +3

±1 = 68%

±2 = 95.45%

±3 = 99.73%

2)   Answer A:

The median value of a series of numbers is the middle value. 12 is the middle or median value for this set of numbers. The mode is 8, which was selection "B". The average value, or the "mean" for the set is 12.14 which was answer "C" and the range is 11 (19-8) which was answer "D". The mean is derived by adding up the data points, which is 85 and dividing by the number of data points (7), which equals 12.1429.

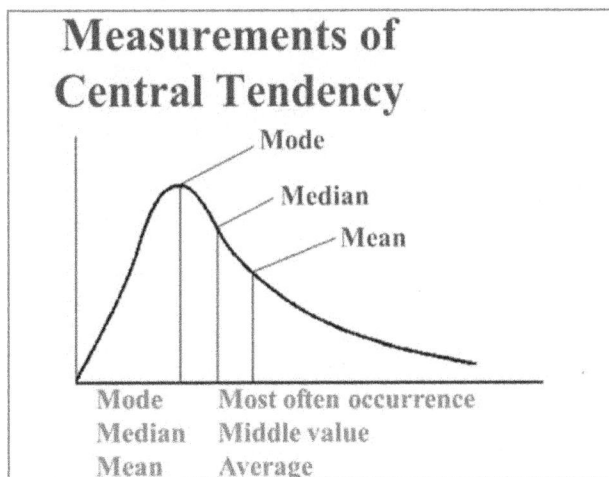

Measurements of Central Tendency

Mode

Median

Mean

Mode	Most often occurrence
Median	Middle value
Mean	Average

3)   Answer D:

System "A" is a parallel system, that is both the first **AND** the second components must fail to produce a system failure. To determine probability for a parallel system, individual probabilities are multiplied.

$$(2 \times 10^{-3}) \times (5 \times 10^{-4}) = 1 \times 10^{-6}$$

System "B" is a series system, that is, if either the first **OR** the second components fail a system failure will occur. For components in series the total failure rate is the sum of individual components' failure rates.

$$(7 \times 10^{-7}) + (3 \times 10^{-7}) = 1 \times 10^{-6}$$

System "C" has only one component. Thus, the probability of system failure is the same as single component probability of failure.

$$1 \times 10^{-6}$$

Since the severity and probability for each system is the same, the loss risk is also the same. Given this situation, the selection process would consider overall system cost, deliverability, quality, longevity, human factors, etc.

4)   Answer C:

During the first random selection you have two chances in 12 of selecting, but in the second selection you only have one chance in 11 in selecting a female.

Probability

$$\text{Probability} = \frac{\text{Number of times event occurs}}{\text{Total number of possible outcomes}}$$

OR

- Work in the probability of Failure
- Draw a fault tree
- Apply the Boolean Logic

Increase knowledge

$$P_{(2 \text{ Female})} = \frac{2}{12} \times \frac{1}{11} = \frac{1}{66} = 0.015$$

Probability

When flipping of a coin:

The probability of getting heads on one toss:

$$P_{HEADS} = \frac{1}{1+1} = \frac{1}{2}$$

The probability of getting 5 in one role of a die:

$$P_{(5)} = \frac{1}{1+1+1+1+1+1} = \frac{1}{6}$$

Probability

The probability of getting twelve when rolling two dice:

$$P_{(12)} = \frac{1}{6} \times \frac{1}{6} = \frac{1}{36}$$

5)   Answer D:

Probability is the number of fork truck accidents divided by the number of total accidents.

$$P = \frac{3}{50} = 0.06 = 6\%$$

6)   Answer B:

Vehicle accident rates are computed to indicate frequency per 1,000,000 miles, therefore:

$$\frac{25 \times 1,000,000}{2,000,000} = 12.5 \text{ accidents per million miles}$$

Note: Be careful - do not confuse the exposure figures. Vehicle accidents are generally measured per million miles, whereas injury rates are figured per 200,000 work hours or 100 workers working one year.

7)   Answer C is correct:

Since profit on the production on the direct cost is 2.5%, there must be a volume of $3,600,000 to cover the workman's compensation losses.

$$90,000 \div .025 = 3,600,000$$

8)   Answer B:

Cost per year = $12,250 ÷ 4 = $3062.50
Cost per month = $3062.50 ÷ 12 = $255.21
Months to recover cost = $30,000.00 ÷ $255.21 = 117.55

9)   Answer A:

The formula to calculate **incident rate** is Recordable accidents times 200,000 divided by the total hours worked. This formula yields the rate of injuries per hundred workers.

$$\text{Rate} = \frac{\text{Total Recordables} \times 200,000}{\text{Total hours}}$$

$$\text{Rate} = \frac{40 \times 200,000}{1,500,000}$$

$$\text{Rate} = 5.33$$

10)   Answer A:

Step 1.   Solve for yearly loss

$$3x = 45,000$$
$$x = \frac{45,000}{3}$$
$$x = 15,000$$

Step 2.   Multiply by 12
$$x = 15,000$$
$$12x = 180,000$$

11)   Answer D:

Step 1.   Solve for yearly loss
$$3x = 90,000$$
$$x = \frac{90,000}{3}$$
$$x = 30,000$$

Step 2.   Multiply by 12
$$x = 30,000$$
$$12x = 360,000$$

Domain 1: Hazard Identification and Control

Domain 1 *Hazard Identification and Control (includes Health Hazards) • 57.1 %*

Knowledge of:

1. Common hazards and controls associated with hot work (e.g., cutting, welding, grinding)
2. Common electrical hazards and controls
3. Common hazards and controls associated with excavations
4. Common hazards and controls associated with working at heights (e.g., ladders, scaffolding, aerial platforms)
5. Common hazards and controls associated with working in confined spaces
6. Common struck by hazards and associated controls
7. Common caught-in or caught-between hazards and associated controls
8. Common hazards and controls associated with hoisting and rigging
9. Common hazards and controls associated with crane operations
10. Common hazards and controls associated with material handling
11. Common hazards and controls associated with material storage
12. Common hazards and controls associated with housekeeping
13. Common hazards and controls associated with powder actuated tools
14. Common hazards and controls associated with hand and power tools
15. Common hazards and controls associated with asbestos exposure
16. Common hazards and controls associated with lead exposure
17. Common hazards and controls associated with noise exposure
18. Common hazards and controls associated with radiation exposure (ionizing and non-ionizing)
19. Common hazards and controls associated with silica exposure
20. Common hazards and controls associated with chemical exposure
21. Common hazards and controls associated with working in extreme temperatures
22. Common hazards and controls associated with vibration and impact exposures
23. The Globally Harmonized System of Classification and Labeling of Chemicals (GHS)
24. Basic safety through design (e.g., incorporating hierarchy of controls into design of building or systems)
25. Risks associated with multiple trades working simultaneously in work area (e.g., congested area, overlapping of workers)
26. Principles of ergonomics as applied to construction practices and material handling
27. Requirements, usage, and limitations of personal protective equipment
28. Basic testing and monitoring equipment (e.g., electrical, industrial hygiene, four gas meter) required for a situation

Skill to:

1. Apply the hierarchy of controls
2. Verify corrective actions were effective in eliminating or mitigating hazards
3. Recognize and address hazards over changing construction site conditions (e.g., excavations after weather events, changing site entrances)
4. Develop job/hazard safety analyses
5. Prioritize identified hazards based on level of risk (e.g., order of severity, probability, frequency)

Hazard Identification and Risk Assessment

Risk assessment is the process to determine the level of risk based on the likelihood the hazard will cause injury or illness, and the severity of the injury or illness that may result. When a hazard is identified and he potential for harm is discussed, and the probability an incident or exposure can occur, a risk assessment has been conducted. For less complex hazards and risks, the assessment may be based entirely on knowledge and experience. The following definitions are from the ANSI Z10-2012, Occupational Health and Safety Management Systems.

- **Hazard:** A condition, set of circumstances, or inherent property that can cause injury, illness, or death.
  Exposure: Contact with or proximity to a hazard, taking into account duration and intensity.
- **Risk:** An estimate of the combination of the likelihood of an occurrence of a hazardous event or exposure(s), and the severity of injury or illness that may be caused by the event or exposures
- **Probability:** The likelihood of a hazard causing an incident or exposure that could result in harm or damage-for a
  selected unit of time, events, population, items or activity being considered.
- **Severity:** The extent of harm or damage that could result from a hazard-related incident or exposures.
- **Risk assessment:** Process(es) used to evaluate the level of risk associated with hazards and system issues.

Risk assessment outcomes are used to determine the relative levels of occupational risk and the importance of developing strategies for risk reduction. It is generally acknowledged that zero risk is practically unattainable and a certain measure of residual risk always remains.

"Safe" can be interpreted as having reached a level of acceptable or minimal residual risk. By identifying acceptable levels of risk, management can best operationalize risk reduction strategies.

According to ANSI Z10, the following represents a general process of risk assessment:

- Assure Management commitment, involvement and direction
- Select a risk assessment team, including employees with knowledge of jobs and tasks.
- Establish the analysis parameters.
- Select a risk assessment technique.
- Identify the hazards.
- Consider failure modes.
- Assess the severity of consequences.
- Determine occurrence probability, prominently taking into consideration the exposures.
- Define the initial risk.
- Make risk acceptance or non-acceptance decisions with employee involvement.
- If needed, select and implement hazard avoidance, elimination, reduction and control measures.
- Address the residual risk.
- Make risk acceptance or non-acceptance decisions with employee involvement.
- Document the results.
- Follow-up on the actions taken.

The goal of a risk assessment process is to achieve safe working conditions with an acceptable level of risk. There is no single, absolute definition for acceptable risk and it will vary by organization. In general terms, acceptable risk is risk that has been assessed and controlled to a level that is tolerated by the organization. Obtaining zero risk is nearly impossible as there is always residual risk when operations continue.

There are a number of risk assessment techniques and the method depends on the complexity of the situation.

Risk assessments may include:

- **Accident/incident investigation**: Although reactive it is another tool for uncovering hazards and management system failures. The primary purpose of the accident/incident investigation is to prevent future occurrences. Therefore, the results of the investigation should be used to initiate corrective action.

- **Brain Storming:** A free flowing group discussion by employees who perform a task to identify hazards, risks, and solutions.

- **Job Safety Analysis** (Job Hazard Analysis): A method that can be used to identify, analyze and record the steps involved in performing a specific job; the existing or potential safety and health hazards associated with each step; and the recommended action(s)/procedure(s) that will eliminate or reduce these hazards and the risk of a workplace injury or illness.

- **Trend Analysis:** Worksite Analysis is analysis of injury and illness trends over time, so that patterns with common causes can be identified and prevented. Review of the OSHA injury and illness forms is the most common form of pattern analysis, but other records of hazards can be analyzed for patterns. Examples are inspection records and employee hazard reporting records.

- **What-if:** For relatively uncomplicated processes, review the process from raw materials to product. At each handling or processing step, "what if" questions are formulated and answered, to evaluate the effects of component failures or procedural errors on the process.

- **Checklist**: For more complex processes, the "what if" study can be best organized through the use of a "checklist," and assigning certain aspects of the process to the committee members having the greatest experience or skill in evaluating those aspects. Operator practices and job knowledge are audited in the field, the suitability of equipment and materials of construction is studied, and the chemistry of the process and the control systems are reviewed, and the operating and maintenance records are audited. Generally, a checklist evaluation of a process precedes use of the more sophisticated methods described below, unless the process has been operated safely for many years and has been subjected to periodic and thorough safety inspections and audits.

- **What-If/Checklist:** The what-if/checklist is a broadly based hazard assessment technique that combines the creative thinking of a selected team of specialists with the methodical focus of a prepared checklist. The result is a comprehensive hazard analysis that is extremely useful in training operation personnel on the hazards of the particular operation.
- **Failure modes and effects analysis (FMEA):** System analysis technique that identifies the manner in which failures occur and investigates their impact on one another, as well as on other parts of the system.
- **Fault-tree analysis (FTA):** System safety technique using deductive (general to specific) analysis that starts with an undesired event and analyzes the way the undesired event can occur. Uses Boolean algebra to simplify the fault-tree diagram to a minimal cut set, which is the shortest, most direct path that allows an event to take place.
- **Hazard and operability study (HAZOP):** Study used to identify problems associated with potential hazards and deviations in plant operations from the design specifications and is carried out by a multidisciplinary team following a structure that includes a series of guide words.
- **Management oversight and risk tree (MORT):** Analytical system that develops a logic tree to identify total system risks, both those inherent in physical equipment and processes and those arising from operational/management inadequacies.
- **Preliminary hazard analysis (PHA):** System safety technique that is the initial effort to identify potentially hazardous components within a system during the design phase.
- **Systems hazard analysis (SHA):** Method that seeks to identify physical and functional incompatibilities between adjacent, interconnected, and interacting elements.
- **System safety engineering report (SSER):** Report that consists of a compilation of the production phase inputs that identifies and documents the hazards of the final product or system and provides definite conclusions about the safety integrity of the product and the manner in which specific hazards have been controlled.

- **System safety program plan (SSPP):** Plan that identifies the tasks to be accomplished in the total safety program for the evolution of the system and is considered the key to a successful program.
- **Technique of human rate error prediction (THREP):** System safety technique that calculates the probability of human operating errors.

Hazard Identification and Assessment

Source	Description
Equipment and machinery manufacturers	Owner and operator manuals typically include (1) warnings of hazards that may be present during operation and instructions, and (2) precautions for safely operating the equipment or machinery.
Chemical manufacturers	Chemical manufacturers are required to provide downstream users with Safety Data Sheets (SDSs). These summarize information about health hazards, and provide instructions on how to safely handle and use the chemical.
Trade associations, insurance carriers, manufacturers, and government agencies	Some trade associations and insurance carriers publish safety and health information. Some manufacturers, and government agencies such as OSHA, the National Institute for Occupational Safety and Health (NIOSH), issue safety and health warnings and hazard alerts directed toward particular products, work practices, or hazards.
Workplace injury and illness information	Data and reports on occupational injuries, illnesses, and fatalities that have occurred in the workplace provide direct evidence of the presence and seriousness of hazards. Most employers are required to maintain logs and summaries of "recordable" occupational injuries and illnesses and to report incidents to OSHA. Incident investigations can uncover previously undetected hazards and ineffective control measures.
Employee safety and health complaints	Employees have first-hand familiarity with the hazards at their workplace. Any prior or recent complaints about safety and health conditions, whether formal or informal, point to potential safety and health hazards.
Medical surveillance activities, and employee exposure data	These results can alert employers to hazards posed by chemical, physical, and biological agents. Use of aggregated results is important to maintain the confidentiality of employee medical information.
Disaster preparedness scenarios	Conducting a "what-if" analysis of possible natural and man-made disasters can help identify hazards that have a low probability of occurrence, but that may have disastrous consequences. Examples include explosions that could be caused by flammable chemicals or combustible dust, hazards that may be created by strong weather phenomena, or incidents related to a criminal or terrorist act.

Hazard Types

Type of Hazard	Source Description and Guidance
Chemical agents	Safety Data Sheets (SDSs) provide a good basis for a developing a list of toxic chemicals in the workplace. When many chemicals are present, hazards of the following types of chemicals should be determined first: chemicals that are (1) volatile; (2) handled or stored in open containers; (3) used in processes where employees are likely to be exposed through inhalation, ingestion, or skin contact; or (4) flammable and stored or used in a manner that poses a fire or explosion hazard.
Biological agents	These include bacteria, viruses, fungi, and other living organisms that can cause acute and chronic infections by entering the body either directly or through breaks in the skin. Sources can include laboratory operations, fermentation processes, or handling of raw food products. They also include exposure to blood or other body fluids or to clients or patients with infectious diseases.
Physical agents	These include excessive levels of ionizing and nonionizing electromagnetic radiation, noise, vibration, illumination, and temperature.
Equipment operation	Ideally, each piece of equipment will be inspected to ensure that all safeguards necessary to protect employees are in place and effective. These include measures to ensure that employees avoid becoming caught in or struck by equipment; burned on hot surfaces; or shocked through contact with energized parts of electric circuits. Important areas of focus for equipment inspection include equipment guarding; the condition of moving parts, parts that support weight, and brakes; and hazards that might arise during maintenance activities
Equipment maintenance	Ideally, the inspection will also include attention to safeguards that ensure that equipment maintenance can be performed safely. This would include such safeguards as deenergizing or otherwise isolating equipment; preventing chemical exposures through appropriate flushing of pumps and other process equipment; releasing stored energy; and use of lockout or tagout to prevent reactivation of equipment during servicing or maintenance.
Fire protection	This part of the inspection would include, for example, making sure that working fire extinguishers are readily available, that flammable liquids and gases are safely handled and stored, and that employees have ready access to emergency exits.
Physical environment	This involves inspecting the facility's walking and working surfaces to identify any trip and fall hazards and ensuring that they are eliminated or controlled.
Work and process flow	The flow of materials and work through an operation can be an important guide to potential hazards. For example, hazards can develop when a product produced at one stage of the process is incompatible with the equipment or practices at the next stage. This could happen in a chemical plant when one piece of equipment produces a hazardous metal catalyst packaged in 55-gallon drums that is then used 5 pounds at a time in another area of the plant. Because of this size difference, employees would need to handle the catalyst manually, causing unnecessary exposures. Producing the catalyst in 5-pound packages would eliminate this hazard.
Work practices	Work practices can be a source of hazards. For example, inappropriate practices for lifting and handling materials can result in back and repetitive motion injuries. When potential hazards are identified, employers can consider whether employees are sufficiently trained to protect themselves. Discussing work practices with employees is particularly important as employees can often identify hazards and solutions based on their day-to-day experience with those practices.

Risk Assessment Matrix

Provides a qualitative method to categorize combinations of indicators and to calculate a risk score.

Likelihood of Occurrence or exposure	Severity and Consequences			
	NEGLIGIBLE: First aid or minor medical treatment	MARGINAL: Minor injury, lost workday	CRITICAL: Disability in excess of 3 months	CATASTROPHIC: Death or permanent total disability
FREQUENT: Likely to occur repeatedly	MEDIUM	SERIOUS	HIGH	HIGH
PROBABLE: Likely to occur several times	MEDIUM	SERIOUS	HIGH	HIGH
OCCASIONAL: Likely to occur sometime	LOW	MEDIUM	SERIOUS	HIGH
REMOTE: Not Likely to Occur	LOW	MEDIUM	MEDIUM	SERIOUS
IMPROBABLE: Very Unlikely to occur	LOW	LOW	LOW	MEDIUM
Risk Level: LOW: Risk acceptable or tolerable, remedial action discretionary. MEDIUM: Take remedial action at appropriate time. SERIOUS: High priority remedial action. HIGH: Operation not permissible. Adapted from ASSE/ANSI Z-10 2012. These definitions are provided for illustration purposes and each organization must define these terms as applicable to their process.				

Hazard Prevention and Control

Some ways to prevent and control hazards are:

- Regularly and thoroughly maintain equipment
- Ensure that hazard correction procedures are in place
- Ensure that everyone knows how to use and maintain PPE
- Make sure that everyone understands and follows safe work procedures

Ensure that, when needed, there is a medical program tailored to your facility to help prevent workplace hazards and exposures.

Engineering Controls

The best strategy after elimination or substitution is to control the hazard at its source. Engineering controls do this, unlike other controls that generally focus on the employee exposed to the hazard. The basic concept behind engineering controls is that, to the extent feasible, the work environment and the job itself should be designed to eliminate hazards or reduce exposure to hazards. Engineering controls can be simple in some cases. They are based on the following principles:

- If feasible, design the facility, equipment, or process to remove the hazard or substitute something that is not hazardous.
- If removal is not feasible, enclose the hazard to prevent exposure in normal operations.
- Where complete enclosure is not feasible, establish barriers or local ventilation to reduce exposure to the hazard in normal operations.

Administrative Controls

Administrative controls are measures aimed at reducing employee exposure to hazards. Safe work practices include your company's general workplace rules and other operation-specific rules. These measures may also include additional relief workers, exercise breaks and rotation of workers. These types of controls are normally used in conjunction with other controls that more directly prevent or control exposure to the hazard

Personal Protective Equipment (PPE)

When exposure to hazards cannot be engineered completely out of normal operations or maintenance work, and when safe work practices and other forms of administrative controls cannot provide sufficient additional protection, a supplementary method of control is the use of protective clothing or equipment. This is collectively called personal protective equipment, or PPE. PPE may also be appropriate for controlling hazards while engineering and work practice controls are being installed.

The basic element of any management program for PPE should be an in depth evaluation of the equipment needed to protect against the hazards at the workplace. The evaluation should be used to set a standard operating procedure for personnel, then train employees on the protective limitations of the PPE, and on its proper use and maintenance.

Using PPE requires hazard awareness and training on the part of the user. Employees must be aware that the equipment does not eliminate the hazard. If the equipment fails, exposure will occur. To reduce the possibility of failure, equipment must be properly fitted and maintained in a clean and serviceable condition

Hierarchy of Controls

The hierarchy provides a systematic way to determine the most effective feasible method to reduce risk associated with a hazard. When controlling the hazard, first consider methods to eliminate the hazard. This is best accomplished in the concept and design phase of a project.

	CONTROLS	EXAMPLES
More Effective	1). Elimination	Design to eliminate hazards: falls, hazardous materials, confined spaces, materials handling, noise, manual handling, etc
	2). Substitution	Substitute for less hazardous materials and equipment, reduce energy, etc.
	3). Engineering Controls	Incorporate safety trough design such as: Ventilation systems, enclosures, guarding, interlocks, lift tables, conveyors, etc.
	4). Warnings	Strategically place signs, alarms, enunciators, labels, etc.
	5). Administrative Controls	Standard Operating Procedures (SOPs) such as: Conduct JSAs, job rotation, inspections, training, mentoring, etc.
Less Effective	6). Personal Protective Equipment	PPE assessments may result in the use of: safety glasses, goggles, face shields, fall protection, protective footwear, gloves, respirators, chemical suits, etc.

Domain 1: Quiz 1 Questions

1). Arrange the following hazard control steps in the proper sequence: (1) guard the hazard (2) engineer the hazard out if possible (3) educate personnel.
   A) 2,1,3
   B) 3,1,2
   C) 1,2,3
   D) 3,2,1

2). The procedure used to make a job safe by identifying hazards in each step of the job and developing measures to counteract those hazards is called:
   A) MORT analysis.
   B) Fault Tree.
   C) Job Safety Analysis.
   D) Probabilistic Risk Assessment.

3). Which of the following reflects the best use of the management tool, Failure Modes and Effects Analysis (FMEA)?
   A) Survey instrument.
   B) Inspection checklist.
   C) Preventative maintenance indicator.
   D) Alternate for fault tree.

4). Which of the following best describes the **evaluation of tasks** involving steps, hazards and solutions?
   A) System Safety Analysis (SSA).
   B) Fault Tree Analysis (FTA).
   C) Job Safety Analysis (JSA).
   D) Management Oversight and Risk Tree (MORT).

5). Which of the following best meets the definition of "Highly Toxic"?
    A) A chemical that causes visible destruction of, or irreversible alterations in, living tissue by chemical action at the site of contact.
    B) A chemical that has a median lethal dose LD 50 of 50 milligrams or less per kilogram of body weight when administered orally to albino rats weighing between 200 and 300 grams each.
    C) A chemical that causes a substantial proportion of exposed people or animals to develop an allergic reaction in normal tissue after repeated exposure to the chemical.
    D) A chemical that has a median lethal dose LD 50 of more than 50 milligrams per kilogram but not more than 500 milligrams per kilogram of body weight when administered orally to albino rats weighing between 200 and 300 grams each.

6). A worker is using a jackhammer with a spade to remove asphalt, what PPE is required?
    A) None, there is not a hazard.
    B) Hearing and eye protection.
    C) Hearing, eye, head and foot protection.
    D) Hearing, eye, head, foot and respiratory protection.

7). Each employee on a walking/working surface (horizontal and vertical surface) with an unprotected side or edge which is ___ feet or more above a lower level shall be protected from falling by the use of guardrail systems, safety net systems, or personal fall arrest systems.
    A) 3
    B) 6
    C) 10
    D) 12

8). Each employee on a scaffold more than ____ feet above a lower level shall be provided with fall protection to prevent from falling to that lower level.
    A) 3
    B) 6
    C) 10
    D) 12

9). The principle value of accident analysis is:
    A) Performance review system.
    B) OSHA reporting system.
    C) Baseline for goals.
    D) Indicator of problem areas.

10). Which of the following diseases would you associate with heavy equipment operators working long hours in cold temperatures?
    A) Brucellosis.
    B) Raynaud's.
    C) Anthrax.
    D) Silicosis.

11). Which of the following is a skin cancer caused by exposure to sunlight?
    A) Mesothelioma.
    B) Sarcomas.
    C) Leukemia.
    D) Melanoma.

12). In order of decreasing effectiveness which of the following correctly indicates the order of corrective actions taken to prevent industrial dermatitis?
    A) Gloves, barrier cream, hygiene.
    B) Substitution, gloves, barrier cream.
    C) Gloves, hygiene, barrier cream.
    D) Substitution, hygiene, barrier cream, gloves.

13). Accidents usually result from:
    A) Personality factors.
    B) Environmental factors.
    C) Physical limitations.
    D) Combinations of factors.

14). Which of the following is the most accurate concerning the listing of a material as a carcinogen on the Safety Data Sheet (SDS)?

A) If there is a report anywhere listing the chemical as a carcinogen then it must be listed as a carcinogen on the SDS.

B) If the substance is identified as an IARC Group 3 or higher it must be listed on the SDS as a carcinogen.

C) If the substance is identified on the National Toxicology Program "Annual Report on Carcinogens" it must be listed on the SDS.

D) If the agent was listed in an in vitro study as a possible group 4 carcinogen risk according to IARC.

15). Which of the following methods is a deductive analysis technique that allows the analyst to determine the combinations of failures that are necessary to achieve an event defined as the top or undesired event?

A) Fault Tree Analysis (FTA).

B) Failure Mode and Effects Analysis (FMEA).

C) Hazard and Operability (HAZOP).

D) Risk Management Plan (RMP).

16). Which of the following provides the best definition of Standard Threshold Shift according to OSHA?

A) An average change in hearing threshold of 5 dB or more at 500, 1000 & 3000 Hz.

B) An average change in hearing threshold of 10 dB or more at 2000, 3000 & 4000 Hz.

C) An average change in hearing threshold of 15 dB or more at 500, 3000 & 6000 Hz.

D) An average change in hearing threshold of 20 dB or more at 2000, 3000 & 4000 Hz.

17). An employee who has experienced a significant threshold shift (STS) is currently working in an area where the Time Weighted Average (TWA) noise level is 100 dBA. If hearing protection is used as the control method, how much attenuation must be provided by the hearing protectors?

A) 10 dB

B) 5 dB

C) 20 dB

D) 15 dB

18). Which of the following methods would be used for determining the uptake of lead in the body of a worker?

A) Expired breath analysis for CO.

B) Blood lead level (PhB) and zinc protoporphyrin (ZPP).

C) Urine for Hippuric Acid.

D) Blood test for cholinesterase activity in red cells.

19). You are reviewing the preliminary plans for the construction of a radio transmitting site located at 9,000 feet elevation. The workers will travel from sea level to the site each day and return after 12-hour shifts. Which of the following would you be most concerned with?

A) Caisson disease.

B) Dequervain's disease.

C) Raynaud's phenomenon.

D) Hypoxia.

20). During a pre-job survey of a sub-contractor's safety program you discover a disturbing program element. The sub-contractor has performed many Job Safety Analyses (JSAs) to satisfy the legal requirement for a hazard analysis, but the JSAs are then filed and never used in the field. All the following are valid uses for a JSA except?

A) To provide training for new workers and refresher training for the old hands.

B) As a survey document when a job or task is modified by new procedures or equipment.

C) As a replacement for job instructions or workplace procedures.

D) As a survey instrument to see if a job has changed since last evaluated and to see if the job is currently being performed correctly.

21). The physiological property of matter that defines the capacity of a chemical to harm or injure a living organism by other than mechanical means is the definition for?

A) Illness.

B) Toxicity.

C) Injury.

D) Pollution.

22). What is this placard?
    A) Flammable liquid.
    B) Flammable solid.
    C) Flammable gas.
    D) Organic peroxide oxidizer.

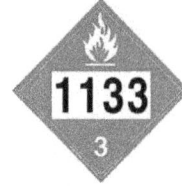

23). A sub-contractor is developing a system safety analysis for the task of dismantling a tower crane attached to the side of a multi-story building. The tower crane will be disassembled, section by section, using a mobile crane. Assuming the analysis will be equipment centered, which system safety analysis technique would be most appropriate for the sub-contractor to use?
    A) Fault Tree Analysis.
    B) Multilinear Events Sequencing.
    C) Job Safety Analysis.
    D) Failure Modes and Effect Analysis.

24). Which system safety tool would be the least effective for analysis of the crane disassembly project described in the last question?
    A) Fault Tree Analysis.
    B) Multilinear Events Sequencing.
    C) Job Safety Analysis.
    D) Failure Modes and Effect Analysis.

25). Which of the following tests/checks would you least expect to be performed during the preparations for disassembly of a tower crane?
    A) Anti-two-block.
    B) Hydraulic.
    C) Non-destructive check of welds.
    D) Automatic fire suppression system.

Domain 1: Quiz 1 Answers

1) Answer A:

Engineering is always the first and most successful method of dealing with a problem. Second choice would be to guard the hazard, and last to educate the human element.

2) Answer C:

The process of Job Safety Analysis examines job hazards during each step of the job and results in improved procedures that almost always increase accident prevention.

3) Answer C:

Preventative maintenance schedules can be developed from the detailed analysis of a system or process that a Failure Mode and Effects Analysis (FMEA) will provide. The analysis provides an indication of which component failure is maintenance dependent as well as how the overall system will benefit from extended life of critical parts.

4) Answer C:

Job Safety Analysis is a systematic analysis of job elements. It results in an in-depth evaluation by workers and first line supervisors of the individual steps and hazards. JSAs also offer protective measures or solutions to identified hazards. Option "A" (System Safety Analysis) is a broad term covering all of the various system safety tools used in the analysis of system risk. Option "B", Fault Tree Analysis is the process of using deductive logic to determine the combination of events that caused a hazardous event to occur. It normally is accompanied by a companion report that evaluates the overall likelihood of failure and provides solutions to the findings discovered in FTA. Option "D" MORT, Management Oversight and Risk Tree is a formal decision tree used in the evaluation of safety programs or as an accident investigation tool. The tool is exhaustive, offering about 1500 events to be evaluated. For this reason it is often considered overkill for all but the largest evaluations or mishaps. However, the system logic is sound and recently several practitioners have produced mini-mort charts that have proven to be useful tools for smaller applications.

5) Answer B:

OSHA at 1910.1200 Appendix A provides definitions for various terms. Selection "A" is the definition of a "Corrosive Chemical". Selection "C" defines a "Sensitizer" and selection "D" provided the definition for "Toxic".

6) Answer C:

Without further information of the actual work conditions, the minimum required would be for hearing, eye, head and foot protection.

1926.95(a)"Application." Protective equipment, including personal protective equipment for eyes, face, head, and extremities, protective clothing, respiratory devices, and protective shields and barriers, shall be provided, used, and maintained in a sanitary and reliable condition wherever it is necessary by reason of hazards of processes or environment, chemical hazards, radiological hazards, or mechanical irritants encountered in a manner capable of causing injury or impairment in the function of any part of the body through absorption, inhalation or physical contact.

7) Answer B:

1926.501(b)(1) "Unprotected sides and edges." Each employee on a walking/working surface (horizontal and vertical surface) with an unprotected side or edge which is 6 feet (1.8 m) or more above a lower level shall be protected from falling by the use of guardrail systems, safety net systems, or personal fall arrest systems.
1926.501(b)(2) "Leading edges": Each employee who is constructing a leading edge 6 feet (1.8 m) or more above lower levels shall be protected from falling by guardrail systems, safety net systems, or personal fall arrest systems. Exception: When the employer can demonstrate that it is infeasible or creates a greater hazard to use these systems, the employer shall develop and implement a fall protection plan which meets the requirements of paragraph (k) of 1926.502. Note: There is a presumption that it is feasible and will not create a greater hazard to implement at least one of the above-listed fall protection systems. Accordingly, the employer has the burden of establishing that it is appropriate to implement a fall protection plan which complies with 1926.502(k) for a particular workplace situation, in lieu of implementing any of those systems. Each employee on a walking/working surface 6 feet (1.8 m) or more above a lower level where leading edges are under construction, but who

is not engaged in the leading edge work, shall be protected from falling by a guardrail system, safety net system, or personal fall arrest system. If a guardrail system is chosen to provide the fall protection, and a controlled access zone has already been established for leading edge work, the control line may be used in lieu of a guardrail along the edge that parallels the leading edge.

8) Answer C:

1926.451(g)(1) – Fall Protection Each employee on a scaffold more than 10 feet (3.1 m) above a lower level shall be protected from falling to that lower level. Paragraphs (g)(1)(i) through (vii) of this section establish the types of fall protection to be provided to the employees on each type of scaffold. Paragraph (g)(2) of this section addresses fall protection for scaffold erectors and dismantlers. Note to paragraph (g)(1): The fall protection requirements for employees installing suspension scaffold support systems on floors, roofs, and other elevated surfaces are set forth in subpart M of this part. Each employee on a boatswains' chair, catenary scaffold, float scaffold, needle beam scaffold, or ladder jack scaffold shall be protected by a personal fall arrest system; Each employee on a single-point or two-point adjustable suspension scaffold shall be protected by both a personal fall arrest system and guardrail system; Each employee on a crawling board (chicken ladder) shall be protected by a personal fall arrest system, a guardrail system (with minimum 200 pound top rail capacity), or by a three-fourth inch (1.9 cm) diameter grab line or equivalent handhold securely fastened beside each crawling board; Each employee on a self-contained adjustable scaffold shall be protected by a guardrail system (with minimum 200 pound top rail capacity) when the platform is supported by the frame structure, and by both a personal fall arrest system and a guardrail system (with minimum 200 pound top rail capacity) when the platform is supported by ropes.

9) Answer D:

The goal of accident analysis is to uncover problem areas.

10) Answer B:

Brucellosis is an infection caused by drinking unpasteurized milk. *Anthrax* is a bacterial infection from animals. *Silicosis* is a *Pneumoconiosis* caused by respirable quartz silica particles hazardous to miners and construction workers. A combination of cold and vibration causes *Raynaud's phenomenon*. This is a condition of the fingers and hands characterized by pallor caused by a diminished blood supply. The disease is most prevalent among workers who use vibrating machinery and are exposed to the cold. Many construction workers encounter these conditions.

11)   Answer D:

Sunlight is the most common occupational cause of melanoma skin cancer.

12)   Answer B:

It is generally accepted within the safety and health industry that substitution is the most effective control method for the prevention of industrial dermatosis. Substitution is followed by gloves and barrier cream. Good hygiene practice is, of course, required in all industrial settings.

13)   Answer D:

Accidents are usually multi-causal in nature and cannot be attributed entirely to any single factor.

14)   Answer C:

OSHA states "Chemical manufacturers, importers and employers evaluating chemicals shall treat the following sources as establishing that a chemical is a carcinogen or potential carcinogen for hazard communication purposes:
- National Toxicology Program (NTP), "Annual Report on Carcinogens" (latest edition)
- International Agency for Research on Cancer (IARC) "Monographs" (latest edition)
- 29 CFR part 1910, subpart Z, Toxic and Hazardous Substances"

Note: The "Registry of Toxic Effects of Chemical Substances" published by the National Institute for Occupational Safety and Health (NIOSH) indicates whether a chemical has been found by NTP or IARC to be a potential carcinogen.

The IARC provides a summary classification of a chemical's carcinogenic risk according to the following table:

Group1   The agent is carcinogenic to humans
Group2A   The agent is probably carcinogenic to humans
Group2B   The agent is possibly carcinogenic to humans
Group3   The agent is not classifiable as to its carcinogenicity to humans
Group4   The agent is probably not carcinogenic to humans

All IARC listed chemicals in Groups 1 and 2A must include appropriate entries on both the SDSs and on the label. Group 2B chemicals need be noted only on the SDSs. The use of in vitro (short term) testing (such as the Ames assay) has not been specifically addressed in the Hazard Communication Standard. However, it is the consensus within OSHA that the results of an "in vitro" test alone, do not represent significant enough information to establish a health hazard for purposes of the hazard communication standard.

15)   Answer A:

Fault Tree Analysis (FTA) is a deductive analysis technique that allows the analyst to determine the combinations of failures that are necessary to achieve an event defined as the top or undesired event. FTA is well suited for the analysis of highly redundant systems. The fault tree is a graphic model that displays the various combinations of equipment/component failures and human errors that can give rise to the top event. The FTA provides a means to qualitatively or quantitatively identify the frequency of the top event. It is a deductive technique that employs Boolean Logic (the use of AND and OR gate logic) to relate the top event to a combination of basic events that must occur in order for the top event to happen. The fault tree, once constructed, can be quantified by using the failure rate data for the basic events (i.e., those events at the bottom of the tree). A quantified fault tree projects the rate of occurrence for the top event.

16)   Answer B:

Standard Threshold Shift (STS) is an indicator of hearing loss that may be revealed by an annual audiogram of an employee. As defined in 29 CFR 1910.95, a standard threshold shift is "a change in hearing threshold relative to the baseline audiogram of an average of 10 dB or more at 2,000, 3,000, and 4,000 Hz in either ear." A Hz is one cycle per second.

17)   Answer D:

For employees who have experienced a significant threshold shift, hearing protector attenuation must be sufficient to reduce employee exposure to a TWA of 85 dB according to OSHA 1910.95.

18)   Answer B:

Biological monitoring for uptake of lead can involve blood lead levels (PhB) and blood zinc protoporphyrin (ZPP), which can show recent uptake. Selection "A" would test for accumulations of carbon monoxide. Selection "C" is the biological marker for exposure to toluene. Selection "D" is a test for exposure to parathion.

19)   Answer D:

Hypoxia is caused by lack of oxygen and can be experienced by industrial workers in extreme elevations under heavy workloads or in confined spaces with oxygen deficiencies. Selection "A", Caisson disease or decompression sickness, could be experienced in divers or other high-pressure environments. One example is underwater tunnels where pressure is maintained to avoid the effects of water leaking into the heading. Selection "B", is a disorder from the narrowing of the tendon sheath for the abductor muscles of the thumb. Dequervain disease is often seen in workers who perform manual tasks requiring firm grips. Selection "C", Raynaud's phenomenon, is sometimes called white finger and results from a combination of cold and vibration.

20)   Answer C:

Job Safety Analysis is a systematic analysis of job elements. It results in an in-depth evaluation by workers and first line supervisors of the individual steps and hazards. JSAs also offer protective measures or solutions to identified hazards. The principle benefits of a Job Safety Analysis (JSA) are:
- Allowing the supervisor to perform training in safe, efficient operations
- Allowing the supervisor or other person developing the JSA to meet and work with employees
- Instruction of new employees on specific jobs
- Instruction of current employees on the specifics of jobs

> performed irregularly
> - As an accident investigation tool should a mishap occur
> - Studying jobs to determine if improvement is possible

21) Answer B:

According to the National Safety Council, "Toxicity is the capacity of a material to produce injury or harm". This differs considerably from the classic definition of hazard, which is the possibility that exposure to a material can cause injury or illness.

22) Answer A:

This placard represents DOT Hazard Class 3, Flammable Liquid. UN1133 is the guide number for Adhesives (flammable).

23) Answer D:

Fault tree analysis is excellent for scaling down huge complex systems, although the tree itself becomes fairly complex. Multilinear Events Sequencing (MES) is an accident investigation tool developed by Ludwig Benner Jr. of the National Transportation Safety Board and used extensively in aircraft mishap investigation. MES is a flow-charting methodology that, as the name implies, puts pertinent events in sequence. The attribute that really makes MES a star performer is the addition of a time line thus allowing duration, interval and sequence dimensions to be visualized. A concept very useful in accident investigation. Failure Modes and Effects Analysis was originally developed to allow predictions for the reliability of complex systems. It uses a tabular format to identify failures and the effect on the overall system. It is an excellent tool for spotting single point failures and would be an excellent choice for this job. Job Safety Analysis is too task oriented to be of much use on this large a job.

24) Answer C:

Of the techniques listed for answers in this question, job safety analysis would be the least effective. JSA tends to be too task oriented to be used successfully in a very complex operation.

25) Answer D:

All the choices would need to be checked if one were to do a thorough analysis. Certainly, one would want to check the anti-two-block prevention device on the mobile crane and inspection of the hydraulic systems would also be a primary consideration. If the crane is used to lift a personnel platform, then an operable anti-two-blocking device is required. Likewise, a check of the welds on each machine is appropriate. We choose the automatic fire suppression system, not because of its importance but because most mobile cranes are not equipped with suppression systems, although engine compartment suppression systems are gaining in popularity on the larger equipment.

Domain 1: Quiz 2 Questions

1) Which of the following is not considered a form of PPE?
    A) Non-slip work boots.
    B) LASER rated safety glasses.
    C) Back Braces.
    D) Face shields.

2) The Safety Data Sheet (SDS) must contain all the following except:
    A) Fire and explosion data.
    B) Health Hazard data.
    C) Protective equipment requirements.
    D) Manufacturer's part number.

3) Which one of the following items is not required on a Hazardous Waste Manifest?
    A) EPA identification number.
    B) Manifest Number.
    C) Liability Insurance Company.
    D) Total quantity of waste shipped.

4) During steel erection, a multiple lift rigging technique is called:
    A) Stack frame erecting.
    B) Pre-cast erecting.
    C) Daisy chaining.
    D) Christmas treeing.

5) The system safety technique that starts with an undesired event and analyzes the way the undesired event occurs is:
    A) The Event Tree.
    B) The Fault Tree.
    C) Known as THERP.
    D) A Job Safety Analysis.

6) Hazard control can be accomplished in a variety of ways. What is the order of precedence of these hazard control methods from highest to lowest?
   A) Using personal protective equipment, designing out the hazard, and eliminating the hazard by substitution or automation, reducing exposure.
   B) Eliminating the hazard by substitution or automation, designing out the hazard, reducing exposure, and using personal protective equipment.
   C) Designing out the hazard, eliminating the hazard by substitution or automation, reducing exposure, and using personal protective equipment.
   D) Designing out the hazard, eliminating the hazard by substitution or automation, using personal protective equipment, and reducing exposure.

7) All the following statements are true concerning the Failure Modes and Effects Analysis (FMEA) except?
   A) FMEA is a reliability tool
   B) FMEA identifies single point failures
   C) FMEA identifies multiple failures, human factors and interfaces
   D) FMEA is normally considered to be inductive

8) Which of the following is an example of pure risk?
   A) Death
   B) Injury that would prevent making a living
   C) A company business failure
   D) Divorce

9) During operations that require a person to be within the control envelope of an industrial robot, a device called a pendant control is used. Which of the following is not true concerning the pendant control?
   A) The pendant has dead man switch provisions
   B) The robot will only operate at slow speed when under pendant control
   C) The pendant control operates in a parallel mode with the master control panel (either can control robot)
   D) The pendant control is equipped with an emergency stop

10) All the following are true concerning the affliction "Metal Fume Fever" except?
   A) MFF is an acute condition of short duration
   B) MFF is a permanent condition, which is compensable thru the workers compensation system in all states
   C) Daily exposure will produce an immunity to MFF
   D) Recovery from MFF is very quick (usually one or two days)

11) The integration of hazard analysis and risk assessment methods early in the design and redesign processes and taking the actions necessary so that the risks of injury or damage are at an acceptable level is termed:
   A) Severity
   B) Prevention through design
   C) Safety through design
   D) Hierarchy of controls

12) Which of the following is a term used to describe the condition "epicondylitis"?
   A) Trigger finger
   B) Rotator cuff
   C) Roofer's wrist
   D) Carpenter's elbow

13) What type of eye protection is required for other workers exposed to welding operations or individuals observing welding operations?
   A) Safety glasses
   B) Goggles with filters
   C) Flame proof screens or goggles
   D) No protections required

14) A major cause of crane fatalities is?
   A) Electrocution
   B) Over turns
   C) Dropped loads
   D) Assembly and dismantling problems

15) When using reinforced concrete and you have rebar protruding from the pour, what is the requirement for fall protection on the rebar?
   A) You are not allowed to have exposed rebar
   B) Cover with plastic caps
   C) Place a plank over the rebar
   D) No protection is required

16) A personal fall arrest system incorporates a body harness requires that the maximum arresting force be limited to:
   A) 900 lbs
   B) 1000 lbs
   C) 1800 lbs
   D) 5000 lbs

17) In some combustible gas meters an electrical circuit called the wheatstone bridge circuit is used to measure the mixture of combustible gas to air. Which of the following characteristics concerning this balanced bridge circuit is not true?
   A) The presence of a combustible mixture causes catalytic combustion decreasing resistance shown as meter movement
   B) One leg of the circuit is called a hot wire
   C) The platinum element can be poisoned by small amounts of silicone
   D) The hot wire detector requires oxygen to function

18) One method of controlling noise is by the use of enclosures. Enclosures are designed to:
   A) Isolate the individual from the noise source
   B) Reduce the noise level at the source
   C) Reduce the internal sound pressure build up
   D) Increase the distance between to source and the receiver

19) Personal protective equipment is very important during welding and cutting operations. Which of the following statements is most correct concerning the proper shade of filter lens to use during welding & cutting operations?
   A) Generally, it is best to pick a #2 lens (dark) and work up, this allows compensation for individual differences
   B) Heavy gas cutting would require a number 6 to 8 shade lens
   C) Heavy gas cutting would require a number 14 to 16 shade lens
   D) As a rule of thumb, it is generally best to start with a lens that gives a clear view of the weld zone and then move up

20) Complete the following statement. A bench grinder should have the tool rest adjusted to within _____ inch of the wheel, and the tongue guard should be adjusted to within _____ inch of the wheel.
   A) 1/2 inch - 1/2 inch
   B) 1/4 inch - 1/8 inch
   C) 1/8 inch - 1/4 inch
   D) 1/16 inch - 1/4 inch

21) Which of the following statements is most correct concerning the use of powder-operated tools in a construction environment?
   A) If a powder-actuated tool misfires, the user must hold the tool in the operating position for at least 30 seconds before trying to fire it again.
   B) Special training is not required for powder-actuated tool operators
   C) Compressed air must be reduced to 30 psi for powder actuated tools
   D) Only specially marked intrinsically safe powder actuated tools may be used in an explosive or flammable atmosphere.

22) The following code is found on your safety shoes, what does the "FI/75" indicate?

ANSI Z41 PT 91
FI/75 C/75 MT/75
Cd 1 EH
PR

   A) Female with an impact rating of 75 ft-lbs
   B) Fire resistant with an impact rating of 75 ft-lbs
   C) Flame proof with an impact rating of 75 ft-lbs
   D) Size in metrics

23) Which of the following provides the best protection when dealing with hoisting and rigging equipment?
   A) Chains, slings and ropes should be inspected before each job
   B) Hoisting and lifting equipment should be inspected daily
   C) A thorough inspection of all chains in use shall be made every 18 months
   D) The use of wire rope that has been birdcaged is permitted for lifting if provided with crosby clamps every six inches

24) How many cubic feet of fresh air is required for each worker underground?
   A) 400 ft^3
   B) 200 ft^3
   C) 50 ft^3
   D) 100 ft^3

25) You are the safety engineer at a large construction site where an excavation is made in Type A soil using a simple slope for protection. The excavation will be open less than 24 hours and is 10 feet in depth. Which of the following best describes the requirements concerning the horizontal to vertical ratio of the slope?
   A) Maximum allowable slope is ½:1
   B) Maximum allowable slope is ¾:1
   C) Maximum allowable slope is 1½:1
   D) Maximum allowable slope is 3:1

Domain 1: Quiz 2 Answers

1).   Answer C:

Back belts, splints, and braces are not recognized as personal protective equipment. NIOSH has publications about the use of back braces and there is insufficient evidence in the scientific literature to conclude that these devices offer any preventive benefits for low back pain or other musculoskeletal related injuries. The preferred approach to prevention of injuries and illnesses, including back injuries, is to eliminate the hazardous condition in the workplace, primarily through engineering controls. Engineering controls in situations involving lifting might include mechanical assists, adjustment of the height of the surface from which or to which material is lifted, or elimination of unnecessary bending or twisting in the task through workstation and equipment design. When engineering controls are insufficient, administrative controls may be used. In the case of lifting, job redesign could be considered. Training of employees and their supervisors in proper lifting techniques is also important.

2).   Answer D:

The SDS is designed to provide in a concise manner the identification information of a potentially harmful substance together with its hazardous ingredients, physical and chemical characteristics, fire and explosion hazard data, reactivity data, health hazard data, precaution for safe handling/use and control measures. The specific part number of the manufacturer is not required.

3).   Answer C:

A manifest does not require an insurance company number. It does require manifest number, EPA ID number and total quantity of shipped waste.

4).   Answer D:

29 CFR 1926.753(e), *Multiple Lift Rigging Procedure*, is in 1926 Subpart R, *Steel Erection*. During the multiple lift (or "christmas treeing") procedure, the hoisted members need to be attached to the rigging assembly beginning with the topmost attachment. That means that employees have to be under the already attached members while continuing the attachment process. Also, the hoisted members are detached from the assembly beginning with the bottom member, so employees are under the remaining members during the unhooking phase of

the operation (see the description of this process in steel erection in Volume 66 of the *Federal Register* at page 5212, January 18, 2001).

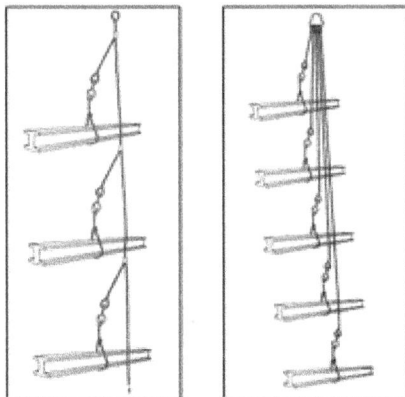

5). Answer B:

A Fault Tree Analysis starts with the undesired event, i.e., the FAULT.

6). Answer C:

Common methods of hazard control include: using personal protective equipment, reducing exposure, designing out the hazard and eliminating the hazard by substitution or automation. According to the National Safety Council Publication *Basics of Safety and Health,* common methods of hazard control, in order of precedence, are: designing out the hazard, eliminating the hazard by substitution or automation, reducing exposure, and using personal protective equipment.

7). Answer C:

The Failure Modes and Effects Analysis (FMEA) is a systematic evaluation of the different ways each individual component can fail and the effects of that failure on the overall system or process. It is generally considered a reliability tool. It does an excellent job of identifying single point failures and is an inductive analysis. The FMEA does not do a good job of identifying failures in complex systems requiring multiple operational interfaces, or multiple failures and it does not address human factors.

Note: If the FMEA is done on a higher level than individual components, which is at a functional level to include groups of components, it can be deductive.

This "Functional FMEA" asks what the cause of the subsystem or assembly level failure might be. It does not assign probability or reliability calculations and is gaining popularity as a deductive system safety tool.

8). Answer A:

Pure risk is a event of failure from which there is no possible recovery. The only example cited is that of death and then only if viewed from a personal viewpoint.

9). Answer C:

The purpose of a pendant control is to allow hands-on control of the robot when programming, teaching, or performing maintenance. Accordingly, the pendant must be the only control device operable when it is being used. Normally it is hardwired to the drive power source rather than through the computer I/O port. The pendant should also contain a dead man switch provision and if two persons are in the primary hazard zone each should be equipped with a dead man switch. Sometimes these additional switches are called enabling devices and have no other function than to stop the action of the robot when released. The pendant cannot operate the robot other than in a slow or crawl mode. A review of robot primary safeguards would be appropriate prior to the examination.

10). Answer B:

Metal Fume Fever (MFF) is an acute affliction that produces flu like symptoms (fever and chills). Recovery is normally complete within one to two days. Daily exposure will cause an immunity, however any disruption such as a weekend off will result in reoccurrence of the symptoms, usually with greater severity. **The cause of MFF is almost always inhalation of high concentrations of zinc oxide fumes.** But there are instances arising from exposure to magnesium oxide and copper oxides.

11). Answer C:

Safety through design is defined as the integration of hazard analysis and risk assessment methods early in the design and redesign processes and taking the actions necessary so that the risks of injury or damage are at an acceptable level. This concept encompasses facilities, hardware, equipment, tools, materials, layout and configuration, energy controls, environmental concerns and products. **Severity.** The extent of harm or damage that could result from. **Prevention through design.** Addressing occupational safety and health needs in the design and redesign processes to prevent or minimize the work-related hazards and risks associated with the construction, manufacture, use, maintenance, and disposal of facilities, materials, equipment and processes. **Hierarchy of controls is a** systematic way of thinking and acting, considering steps in a ranked and sequential order, to choose the most effective means of eliminating or reducing hazards and the risks that derive from them. An example is the requirement of suppliers of services to attest that processes have been applied to identify and analyze hazards and to reduce the risks deriving from those hazards to an acceptable level. Manufacturers of equipment to be used in the European Union are required by International Organization for Standardization (ISO) standards to certify that they have met applicable standards, including ISO 12100-1 and ISO 14121.]

12).   Answer D:

The disorder "epicondylitis" is often called tennis elbow or sometimes carpenter's elbow. The disorder is a result of combined motion causing pronation of the hand and ulnar deviation. For a carpenter this involves swinging heavy hammers and in tennis swinging the racket. The affliction causes considerable pain in the hand, forearm and elbow. The term *rotator cuff* is associated with the tearing of a ligament in the shoulder. *Roofer's wrist* is a common name for carpal tunnel syndrome which is a disorder caused by compression of the median nerve. *Trigger finger* is an affliction caused by repeated use of the finger pulling levers or triggers, eg: paint spray operators.

13).   Answer C:

1910.252(b)(2)(i)(A): Helmets or hand shields shall be used during all arc welding or arc cutting operations, excluding submerged arc welding. Helpers or attendants shall be provided with proper eye protection.
1910.252(b)(2)(iii): Protection from arc welding rays. Where the work permits, the welder should be enclosed in an individual booth painted with a finish of low reflectivity such as zinc oxide (an important factor for absorbing ultraviolet radiations) and lamp black or shall be enclosed with noncombustible screens similarly painted. Booths and screens shall permit circulation of air at floor level. Workers or other persons adjacent to the welding areas shall be protected from the rays by noncombustible or flameproof screens or shields or shall be required to wear appropriate goggles.

14). Answer A:

Overhead crane accidents can be attributed to a number of causes. Electrocution is the most common cause of injury in overhead crane accidents. Approximately 40 to 45 percent of all overhead crane accidents involve electrocution that results from the crane contacting a power source during operation. Other major causes of overhead crane accidents include assembly and dismantling problems, falls, crushing by counter weight, dropped loads, outrigger use, crane overturns, boom buckling or collapse, and rigging failure.

15). Answer B:

1926.701(b): Reinforcing steel. All protruding reinforcing steel, onto and into which employees could fall, shall be guarded to eliminate the hazard of impalement. Although "C" may provide protection, the plastic caps designed to cover rebar are considered the best practice in the industry and by OSHA.

16). Answer C:

1926.502(d)(16) also requires that the maximum arresting force be limited to 900 pounds when the personal fall arrest system incorporates a body belt and 1800 pounds when the system incorporates a body harness. If the employer has documentation to demonstrate that these maximum arresting forces are not exceeded and that the personal fall arrest system will operate properly, OSHA will not issue a citation for violation of the free fall distance.

17). Answer A:

Selection "A" is not true. The presence of a combustible mixture causes catalytic combustion on the surface of the hot wire causing an increase in resistance that is converted into a meter movement. The other characteristics of the combustible gas analyzer and the wheatstone bridge circuit are true. A combustible gas monitor is an appropriate instrument when checking concentrations of explosive gases.

18). Answer C:

Generally, an enclosure is placed around a noise source to prevent noise from getting outside. Enclosures are normally lined with sound-absorption material to decrease internal sound pressure buildup.

19).   Answer B:

Proper eye protection is among the most important safety precautions welders and metal cutters can take. The proper shade protection is very important to guard against the damage caused by UV and IR radiation created during these operations. The table shown here was taken directly from the OSHA standards. Additional information is contained in ANSI/ASC Z49.1-88.

OSHA 1926.102 Table E-2
FILTER LENS SHADE NUMBERS FOR PROTECTION AGAINST RADIANT ENERGY

Welding Operation	Shade Number
Shielded metal-arc welding 1/16, 3/32, 1/8, 5/32 inch diameter electrodes	10
Gas-shielded arc welding (nonferrous) 1/16, 3/32, 1/8, 5/32 inch diameter electrodes	11
Gas-shielded arc welding (ferrous) 1/16, 3/32, 1/8, 5/32 inch diameter electrodes	12
Shielded metal-arc welding 3/16, 7/32, 1/4 inch diameter electrodes	12
5/16, 3/8 inch diameter electrodes	14
Atomic hydrogen welding	10-14
Carbon-arc welding	14
Soldering	2
Torch brazing	3 or 4
Light cutting, up to 1 inch	3 or 4
Medium cutting, 1 inch to 6 inches	4 or 5
Heavy cutting, over 6 inches	5 or 6
Gas welding (light), up to 1/8 inch	4 or 5
Gas welding (medium), 1/8 inch to 1/2 inch	5 or 6
Gas welding (heavy), over 1/2 inch	6 or 8

20). Answer C:

According to the National Safety Council's "Accident Prevention Manual for Industrial Operations." Tool rests should be adjusted to not more than 1/8 inch from the grinding wheel, tongue guards should be adjusted to 1/4 inch.

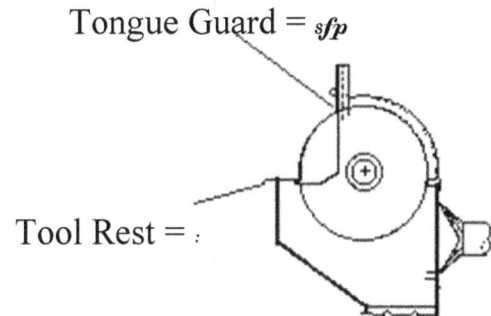

Tongue Guard = *sfp*

Tool Rest = *

21). Answer A:

Powder-actuated tools operate like a loaded gun and must be treated with extreme caution. In fact, they are so dangerous that they must be operated only by specially trained employees. When using powder-actuated tools, an employee must wear suitable ear, eye, and face protection. The user must select a powder level -- high or low velocity -- that is appropriate for the powder-actuated tool and necessary to do the work without excessive force. The muzzle end of the tool must have a protective shield or guard centered perpendicular to and concentric with the barrel to confine any fragments or particles that are projected when the tool is fired. A tool containing a high-velocity load must be designed not to fire unless it has this kind of safety device. To prevent the tool from firing accidentally, two separate motions are required for firing. The first motion is to bring the tool into the firing position, and the second motion is to pull the trigger. The tool must not be able to operate until it is pressed against the work surface with a force of at least 5 pounds (2.2 kg) greater than the total weight of the tool. If a powder-actuated tool misfires, the user must hold the tool in the operating position for at least 30 seconds before trying to fire it again. If it still will not fire, the user must hold the tool in the operating position for another 30 seconds and then carefully remove the load in accordance with the manufacturer's instructions. This procedure will make the faulty cartridge less likely to explode. The bad cartridge should then be put in water immediately after removal. If the tool develops a defect during use, it should be *tagged* and must be *taken out of service immediately* until it is properly repaired. Safety precautions that must be followed when using powder-actuated tools include the following:

- Do not use a tool in an explosive or flammable atmosphere.
- Inspect the tool before using it to determine that it is clean, that all moving parts operate freely, and that the barrel is free from obstructions

and has the proper shield, guard, and attachments recommended by the manufacturer.

- Do not load the tool unless it is to be used immediately.
- Do not leave a loaded tool unattended, especially where it would be available to unauthorized persons.
- Keep hands clear of the barrel end.
- Never point the tool at anyone.

When using powder-actuated tools to apply fasteners, several additional procedures must be followed:

- Do not fire fasteners into material that would allow the fasteners to pass through to the other side.
- Do not drive fasteners into very hard or brittle material that might chip or splatter or make the fasteners ricochet.
- Always use an alignment guide when shooting fasteners into existing holes.
- When using a high-velocity tool, do not drive fasteners more than 3 inches (7.62 centimeters) from an unsupported edge or corner of material such as brick or concrete.
- When using a high velocity tool, do not place fasteners in steel any closer than $^1/2$-inch (1.27 centimeters) from an unsupported corner edge unless a special guard, fixture, or jig is use

22). Answer A:
The protective identification ANSI code will be legible (printed, stitched, etc.) on one shoe of each pair. The following is an example of an ANSI code on a piece of protective footwear:

ANSI Z41 PT 91
FI/75 C/75 MT/75
Cd 1 EH
PR

Line #1: ANSI Z41 PT91. This line identifies the ANSI Z41 standard. The letters PT indicates the protective section of the standard. This is followed by the last two digits of the year of the standard with which the footwear meets compliance (1991)
Line #2: FI/75 C/75 MT/75. This line identifies the applicable gender (M or F) for which the footwear is intended. It also identifies the existence of impact resistance (I), the impact resistance rating (75, 50, or 30 foot-pounds). This line can also include a metatarsal protection designation (MT) and rating (75, 50, or 30 foot-pounds).

Lines #3 & 4: Cd 1 EH; PR. This area of the label designates conductive properties (Cd) and type (1 or 2), electrical hazard (EH) and puncture resistance (PR), if applicable.

23).   Answer A:

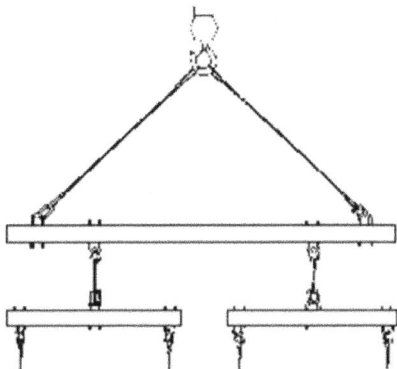

Inspection of hoisting and rigging equipment before each job provides the greatest protection from use of defective equipment. Selection "B" is a good practice, however not as protective as choice "A". The frequency on selection "C" should be dependent on use, however in no case more than 12 months. Selection "D" is incorrect, bird-caged wire rope should be removed from service. **1926.502(d)(21)** Personal fall arrest systems shall be inspected prior to each use for wear, damage and other deterioration and defective components shall be removed from service.

24).   Answer B:

To prevent any dangerous or harmful accumulation of dusts, fumes, mists, vapors, or gases OSHA 1926.800(k)(1)(ii)(2) requires a minimum of 200 cubic feet of fresh air per minute to be supplied for each employee underground.

25). Answer A:

OSHA 1926, Subpart P, Appendix B requires an excavation in Type A soil that is open less than 24 hours and is 12 feet or less in depth to have a maximum allowable slope of ½:1.

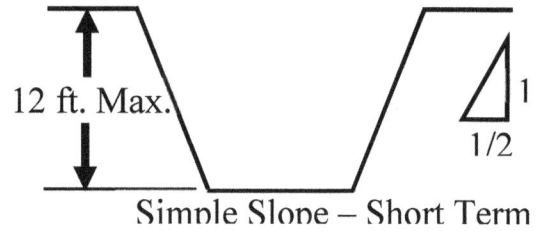

12 ft. Max.

1

1/2

Simple Slope – Short Term

Domain 1: Quiz 3 Questions

1). An excavation is made in Type C soil using a simple slope for protection. The excavation will be open for greater than 36 hours and is 14 feet in depth. Which of the following best describes the requirements concerning the horizontal to vertical ratio of the slope?
    A) Maximum allowable slope is ½:1
    B) Maximum allowable slope is ¾:1
    C) Maximum allowable slope is 1½:1
    D) Maximum allowable slope is 3:1

2). Which of the following items of test equipment would be the most accurate in measuring the *amount* of resistance in an equipment ground?
    A) Lamp and battery.
    B) Battery and buzzer/bell.
    C) Neon lamp.
    D) Ground loop impedance tester.

3). Which of the following instruments would be the best selection to check the conductivity of the case ground (green wire) connection on a portable hand held electric drill.
    A) Split core ammeter.
    B) Megger.
    C) Volt-ohm meter.
    D) Ground loop impedance tester with auxiliary tension device.

4). Which of the following is not true concerning the electrical Ground Fault Circuit Interrupter?
    A) It requires an equipment ground to function.
    B) It is a very fast acting device.
    C) It will not detect line-to-line faults.
    D) It is designed for personnel protection.

5). One of the problems associated with arc welding of stainless steel is the production of aerosols containing:
    A) Nickel and Chromium.
    B) Carbon and Nickel.
    C) Fluorides, Nickel and Chromium.
    D) Copper, Nickel and Acid gases.

6). Which of the following trades would most likely be exposed to the damaging effects of fluorides?
   A) Welder.
   B) Stone Mason.
   C) Laborer.
   D) Carpenter.

7). At what depth must a trench be provided with means of egress such as a stairway, ladder, ramp etc.?
   A) Greater than 8 feet.
   B) 5 feet or more.
   C) 4 feet or more.
   D) 16 feet or more.

8). An overhead crane is equipped with a hoist line limit switch. The purpose of this device is?
   A) To prevent the crane from lifting a weight beyond the load limit.
   B) To prevent the load from being lifted too fast.
   C) To prevent over travel of the load block.
   D) To prevent the crane magnet from being disconnected during lifting.

9). When supplying breathing air to five or more abrasive blasting respirators, what is the minimum amount of air to be supplied to each unit?
   A) 3 CFM
   B) 6 CFM
   C) 9 CFM
   D) 12 CFM

10). The hoods on grinders and cutting wheels establish the platform for a tongue guard that must be placed within 1/4 inch of the periphery of the wheel. The hood also serves several other purposes including:
   A) Removal of dust and dirt generated by the operation.
   B) Covering at least 85% of the wheel.
   C) Providing protection from falling into the wheel.
   D) Removal of particles and shielding operator from hazard if wheel should break.

11). When using a powered woodcutting "table" saw which of the following would have the least effect on either causing or preventing kickbacks?
   A) Maintaining the rip fence parallel to the saw blade.
   B) Installing and maintaining a spreader.
   C) Ripping work that is twisted or warped.
   D) Removing blade cover guard.

12). Which of the following electrical devices would most likely contain polychlorinated biphenyl (PCBs)?
   A) Transformers, capacitors, fluorescent light ballasts.
   B) Fuses, wiring and meters.
   C) Circuit breakers, panel board and Unistrut.
   D) Meters, relays and switches.

13). Which of the following best describes a Class "B" level of Personal Protective Equipment (PPE)?
   A) Fully-encapsulated chemical-resistant suit with Self Contained Breathing Apparatus (SCBA) or Supplied Air (SA) with escape provisions.
   B) Chemical-resistant suit with Self Contained Breathing Apparatus (SCBA) or Supplied Air (SA) with escape provisions.
   C) Chemical-resistant suit with Air Purifying Respirator (APR).
   D) No chemical protection and no respiratory protection.

14). American National Standard Z89.1-1997 establishes specifications for helmets (hardhats) to protect the heads of industrial workers from impact and penetration by falling objects and from high-voltage electrical shock. Which of the following classes offers low voltage protection?
   A) A
   B) C
   C) E
   D) G

15). At what depth must a trench be shored or cut to the angle of repose?
   A)   Greater than 4 feet.
   B)   5 feet or more.
   C)   4 feet.
   D)   6 feet or more.

16). If a person is suffering from heatstroke, which symptom would they not experience?
- A) Severe headache.
- B) Profuse sweating and cool moist skin.
- C) Loss of consciousness.
- D) Rapid temperature rises and hot dry skin.

17). Which of the following is only an internal radiation hazard?
- A) Alpha.
- B) Beta.
- C) Gamma or X-Ray.
- D) Neutron.

18). If variations in noise levels are occurring at a rate more often than once per second, the noise is considered _____.
- A) Impulse.
- B) Impact.
- C) Continuous.
- D) Sporadic.

19). Which of the following heat stress indicators is most commonly used in the Health & Safety field?
- A) Effective Temperature.
- B) Belding Hatch Stress Index.
- C) Wet Bulb Globe Thermometer Index.
- D) Skin Wetness.

20). Which of the following is the most effective method of preventing inadvertent startup of electrical equipment that may cause injury or property damage?
- A) Tagout.
- B) Enclosure.
- C) Lockout.
- D) Warning Signs.

21). What are the axes of a conventional risk matrix?
- A) Risk *vs.* Likelihood.
- B) Number of Loss Scenarios vs. Probability.
- C) Likelihood vs. Consequence.
- D) Severity vs. Magnitude.

22). During a forklift operation at your site you observe the back of a rough terrain forklift tip as a heavy load is being lifted. Which of the following is the proper course of action?

    A) Add extra counter weight to stabilize the operation.
    B) Do not continue with this lift.
    C) Add air to the load side tires.
    D) Tip the mast back once the load is lifted.

23). Guardrail systems shall be capable of withstanding, without failure, a force of at least _____ pounds applied within 2 inches (5.1 cm) of the top edge, in any outward or downward direction, at any point along the top edge.

    A) 150 pounds.
    B) 200 pounds.
    C) 210 pounds.
    D) 240 pounds.

24). Many workplaces contain areas that are considered "confined spaces" A confined space has limited or restricted means for entry or exit, not designed for continuous occupancy and;

    A) Has a potentially hazardous atmosphere.
    B) Are large enough for workers to enter and perform work.
    C) Has an engulfment or entrapment configuration.
    D) Are large enough for the body to pass the plane of the opening.

25). Which of the following would be the hardest to remove during decontamination?

    A) Chemical permeated into PPE material.
    B) Dried solid materials caked onto PPE.
    C) Liquid material spread into crevices and pleats of the PPE.
    D) Sludges splattered onto the PPE

Domain 1: Quiz 3 Answers

1). Answer C:

OSHA 1926, Subpart P, Appendix B requires an excavation in Type C soil that is 20 feet or less in depth to have a maximum allowable slope of 1½:1.

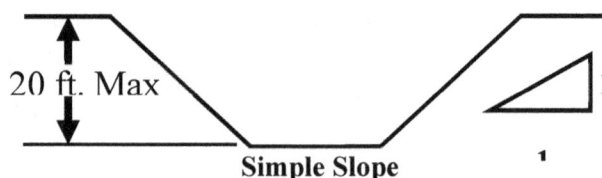

20 ft. Max

Simple Slope

1

2). Answer D:

The requirements for an Assured Equipment Grounding Conductor Program are contained in 29 CFR 1926.404. This standard requires a written description of the employer's assured equipment grounding conductor program, including the specific procedures to be used, be kept at the jobsite. Additionally, testing must be done to determine the continuity of the equipment grounding conductor and to ensure the correct polarity of receptacles and plugs.

Of the equipment listed only the ground impedance tester would indicate the amount of resistance presented to current flow by the equipment ground. All of the other devices would provide an indication of continuity not amount of resistance. An additional piece of equipment that could be used to indicate the amount of resistance would have been the standard volt-ohm meter. However, the difference between the volt-ohm-meter and the ground impedance meter is significant. Impedance checking devices provide information about both high and low current ground faults, whereas the standard volt-ohm-meter would only tell us about protection from low current faults. OSHA at 1910.404 requires two tests. One is a continuity test to ensure that the equipment grounding conductor is electrically continuous. It is performed on all cord sets, receptacles etc. which are not part of the permanent wiring of the structure. The test may be performed, according to OSHA, using a simple continuity tester such as a lamp and battery, a bell and battery, an ohmmeter, or a receptacle tester. The other test required by OSHA is a polarity check on receptacles and plugs to make sure that the equipment grounding conductor is connected to the correct terminal. The same simple equipment used for the continuity test can be used for this test.

3). Answer C:

Most hand-held equipment in use today is of the double insulated type and therefore does not require a third wire. However, the standard volt-ohm meter would do an acceptable job of checking the continuity of the case ground on a portable electrical drill. Selection "A" the split core ammeter provides a safe way to check amperage on live (hot) circuits. Selection "B" & "D", the megger and ground loop impedance tester are instruments that may be used to check the capability of the equipment ground on a branch circuit within the building or facility.   A ground is an object that connects a piece of electrical equipment to earth or some conducting body that serves in place of the earth. A ground serves to complete the electrical circuit and prevent current from unexpectedly flowing through an individual.

4). Answer A:

The Ground-Fault Circuit Interrupter is a fast-action device that senses a small current leakage to ground and, in a fraction of a second, shuts off the electricity and *interrupts* the faulty flow to ground. Placed between the electrical service and the tool or appliance it serves, the GFCI continually matches the amount of current going to and from the tool along the normal path of the circuit conductors. Whenever the amount *going* differs from the amount *returning* by a set trip level the GFCI interrupts the electric power within 1/40th of a second. This difference in current is called leakage current to ground and the path it takes to ground could be through a person - in which case, the rapid response of the GFCI is fast enough to prevent electrocution. This protection provided by the GFCI is independent of the condition of the equipment grounding conductor, thus, the GFCI can provide protection even if the equipment grounding conductor becomes inoperative. It will however, not detect line-to-line faults.

5). Answer C:

Stainless steel welding results in fumes containing nickel and chromium. The electrodes used in this process often contain large amounts of fluorides that are released into the air in large quantities. According to OSHA at 1910.252, "Brazing and gas welding fluxes containing fluorine compounds shall have a cautionary warning to indicate that they contain fluorine compounds. One such cautionary warning recommended by the American Welding Society for brazing and gas welding fluxes reads as follows:

CAUTION CONTAINS FLUORIDES
This flux when heated gives off fumes that may irritate eyes, nose and throat.

1.   Avoid fumes - use only in well-ventilated spaces.
2.   Avoid contact of flux with eyes or skin.
3.   Do not take internally.

6).   Answer A:

Welders have the potential to be exposed to a variety of health hazards. Among those is fluoride fumes from welding on stainless steel using rods containing fluoride or with some fluxes such as those used in electroslag and submerged arc welding.

7).   Answer C:

Means of egress from trench excavations such as a stairway, ladder, ramp or other safe means of egress are required in trench excavations that are 4 feet or more in depth and located so as to require no more than 25 feet of lateral travel for workers. OSHA 1926.651.

8).   Answer C:

Overhead cranes can be equipped with several types of limit switches. However, the only valid choice in this selection is to prevent the over travel of the load block. This prevents the load block from being drawn into the sheave or drums and is often referred to as an anti-two block device. In the illustration shown here a switch is attached to the crane boom. The switch is held in the closed position by a weight that slides down the hoisting line. When the load block comes too close to the point sheave the weight is lifted and allows the spring-loaded switch to open and disconnect power to the hoist motor.

9).   Answer B:

Respirable air under suitable pressure should be delivered to each respirator at a volume of at least 6 CFM.

10). Answer D:

Hoods on grinding and cutting operations serve a dual function; they protect the worker for the hazards of a bursting wheel, and provide for removal of the dirt, dust and material generated during grinding or cutting operations. Selection "A" is only partially correct. Selection "B" is not correct only 66% of the wheel needs to be covered. Selection "C" is true but is not the best answer.

11). Answer D:

Maintaining the rip fence parallel to the saw blade or installing and maintaining a spreader would tend to prevent kickbacks. Ripping work that is twisted or warped will cause kickbacks. Selection "D" is the best choice, although this is an extremely dangerous practice and should not be permitted, removing the blade cover guard would not have any effect on kickbacks (unless the spreader or anti-kickback dogs are built into the guard). A kickback usually happens during ripping operations when the work is violently thrown back against the operators feeding force.

12). Answer A:

Polychlorinated biphenyl (PCBs) are found in certain electrical devices such as transformers, capacitors, fluorescent light ballasts, etc. as well as in heat transfer enclosures and investment casting waxes in foundries. In 1978, the EPA banned the use of PCBs in light ballasts, transformers and capacitors however it is still possible to find equipment containing PCBs.

13). Answer B:

Modified Chart of EPA/OSHA Levels of Protection			
Levels	Skin	Respiratory	When
A	Fully-encapsulating, chemical-resistant suit, inner gloves, chemical-resistant safety boots.	Pressure-demand, full-facepiece SCBA or pressure-demand supplied-air respirator with escape SCBA.	Highest level of protection indicated by high concentration of atmospheric vapors, gases or particulates or splash hazard exists.
B	Chemical-resistant clothing (overalls and long-sleeved jacket; hooded, one or two piece chemical splash suit; disposable chemical-resistant one-piece suit), inner and outer gloves, chemical resistant safety boots and hard hat.	Pressure-demand, full-facepiece SCBA or pressure-demand supplied-air respirator with escape SCBA.	High level of respiratory protection required, but less skin protection. IDLH, less than 19.5% oxygen.
C	Chemical-resistant clothing (overalls and long-sleeved jacket; hooded, one or two piece chemical splash suit; disposable chemical-resistant one-piece suit), inner and outer gloves, chemical resistant safety boots and hard hat.	Full-facepiece, air-purifying, canister-equipped respirator.	The contaminants, splashes, or direct contact will not affect exposed flesh. Canister will remove contaminant.
D	Overalls, Safety Boots, safety glasses or chemical splash goggles, hardhat.	No respiratory protection and minimal skin protection.	The atmosphere contains no known hazard. Splashes, immersion or inhalation improbable

14). Answer D:

Helmet Types

Class E (Electrical) helmets intended to reduce the danger of exposure to high voltage electrical conductors, proof tested at 20,000 volts. Class E is tested for force transmission first, then tested at 20,000 volts for 3 minutes, with 9 milliamps maximum current leakage; then tested at 30,000 volts, with no burn-through permitted.(formerly Class B)

Class G (General) helmets intended to reduce the danger of exposure to low voltage electrical conductors, proof tested at 2,200 volts. Class G is tested at 2,200 volts for 1 minute, with 3 milliamps max. leakage. (formerly Class A)

Class C (Conductive) helmets not intended to provide protection from electrical conductors. Class C is not tested for electrical resistance. (no change in class designation)

Definitions expanded; new test protocol section, including preparation, mounting, number, and sequence of test samples; summary of failure criteria.
- Product tested within 3 inch circle on top of helmet in "as worn" position
- 2.2 pound pointed steel penetrator, with 60° angle, dropped from a simulated free-fall height of 8 feet
- Penetrator can't make contact w/ head form
- Test apparatus includes electronic contact indicator, velocity indicator, & electronic recording equipment
- No differentiation for helmet classes

15). Answer B:

Excavations that are less than 5 feet in depth do not require shoring or sloping if examination of the ground is conducted by a competent person, who finds no indication of a potential cave-in. The "angle of repose" is the angle at which soil will no longer slide, in this instance it means to slope to a flat enough angle to prevent the soil from sliding back into the ditch. A quick review of OSHA 1926.651 and 652 is in order prior to taking the CHST examination.

16). Answer B:

During heatstroke (sunstroke) the body temperature rises and reaches a point where the heat-regulating mechanism breaks down completely. The body temperature then rises rapidly. The symptoms are hot dry skin, severe headache, visual disturbances, rapid temperature rise, and loss of consciousness.

17). Answer A:

Alpha radiation is non-penetrating and is not considered an external hazard because of the protection provided by the outer layer of skin. Note - in this instance the eyes are considered an internal exposure.

18). Answer C:

If the occurrence of the sound is greater than once per second, the sound is continuous and should be measured as continuous sound. Ref. OSHA 29 CFR 1910.95.

19). Answer C:

The most commonly used heat stress index is the National Institute for Occupational Safety and Health (NIOSH) Wet Bulb Globe Thermometer Index (WBGT).

20). Answer C:

The Control of Hazardous Energy is a fundamental accident prevention control program that affects the control of all potential and kinetic energy (not just electrical). It is addressed in great detail in OSHA at 1910.147. The most effective method of preventing inadvertent startup of equipment is to provide a substantial lock with rigid key control, combined with a tag and education of all personnel involved.

21). Answer C:

According to *Principles of Risk-based Decision Making,* A risk matrix is merely a graphic, or tabular representation of the components of risk itself (e.g frequency/likelihood and consequence/severity).

22). Answer B:

A fork truck should never be operated with an overload. This condition removes weight from the steering wheels, which affects the control of the machine. Never add counterweight because it can seriously overload the forks, tires, axles, chains etc.

23). Answer B:

1926.502(b) "Guardrail systems." Guardrail systems and their use shall comply with the following provisions:
- Top edge height of top rails, or equivalent guardrail system members, shall be 42 inches (1.1 m) plus or minus 3 inches (8 cm) above the walking/working level. When conditions warrant, the height of the top edge may exceed the 45-inch height, provided the guardrail system meets all other criteria of this paragraph.

Note: When employees are using stilts, the top edge height of the top rail, or equivalent member, shall be increased an amount equal to the height of the stilts.

- Midrails, screens, mesh, intermediate vertical members, or equivalent intermediate structural members shall be installed between the top edge of the guardrail system and the walking/working surface when there is no wall or parapet wall at least 21 inches (53 cm) high.
- Midrails, when used, shall be installed at a height midway between the top edge of the guardrail system and the walking/working level.
- Screens and mesh, when used, shall extend from the top rail to the walking/working level and along the entire opening between top rail supports.
- Intermediate members (such as balusters), when used between posts, shall be not more than 19 inches (48 cm) apart.
- Other structural members (such as additional midrails and architectural panels) shall be installed such that there are no openings in the guardrail system that are more than 19 inches (.5 m) wide.
- Guardrail systems shall be capable of withstanding, without failure, a force of at least 200 pounds (890 N) applied within 2 inches (5.1 cm) of the top edge, in any outward or downward direction, at any point along the top edge.

24). Answer B:

"Confined spaces" are defined as:
- large enough for workers to enter and perform certain jobs.
- limited or restricted means for entry or exit and
- is not designed for continuous occupancy.

Confined spaces include, but are not limited to, tanks, vessels, silos, storage bins, hoppers, vaults, pits, manholes, tunnels, equipment housings, ductwork, pipelines, etc. OSHA uses the term "permit-required confined space" (permit space) to describe a confined space that has one or more of the following characteristics: contains or has the potential to contain a hazardous atmosphere; contains material that has the potential to engulf an entrant; has walls that converge inward or floors that slope downward and taper into a smaller area which could trap or asphyxiate an entrant; or contains any other recognized safety or health hazard, such as unguarded machinery, exposed live wires, or heat stress.

25).   Answer A:

Chemical permeated into PPE material is the most difficult to remove. Most PPE manufacturers recommend disposal of permeated PPE.

Domain 1: Quiz 4 Questions

1). Using the chart below determine the Maximum Use Concentration (MUC) for a half-mask respirator with dust/mist filters for Aluminum Metal Dust. The TLV for Aluminum Metal Dust is 10 mg/m^3.

TYPE OF RESPIRATOR	Respirator Assigned Protection Factors		
	Qualitative	Quantitative	IDLH
Particulate-filter, Vapor or gas, quarter or half mask. Includes combination filters.	10	Per-individual max of 100	NO
Particulate-filter, Vapor or gas, full face piece. Includes combination filters.	100	Per-individual max of 100	NO
Powered particulate-filter, Vapor or gas, full face piece any respiratory inlet covering.	No test required due to positive pressure. Max protection is 3000 with high efficiency filter.		NO

        A) 10 mg/m^3
        B) 1 mg/m^3
        C) 100 mg/m^3
        D) 10,000 mg/m^3

2). Which of the following types of radiation from welding operations is the most damaging to the eye?
        A) Light.
        B) Ultraviolet.
        C) Infrared.
        D) Visible light.

3). American National Standard Z89.1-1997 establishes specifications for helmets (hardhats) to protect the heads of industrial workers from impact and penetration by falling objects and from high-voltage electrical shock. Which of the following classes offers high voltage protection?
        A) A
        B) C
        C) E
        D) G

4). Noise measurements produce readings of 84.1 dBC and 84.8 dBA. In which of the following frequency ranges would you most suspect high noise levels?
    A) 50 - 1000
    B) 50 - 500
    C) 500 - 900
    D) 1000 - 3000

5). Which of the following best fits the description of an anti-two block device?
    A) A device installed on an overhead crane to prevent lifting a weight beyond the load limit.
    B) A device designed to keep safety blocks from being inserted into a power press ram control.
    C) A device to prevent over travel of the load block on a mobile crane.
    D) A device that limits the amount of material that can be deposited in the muck bucket attachment on a hoist way man basket.

6). A direct reading instrument indicates a concentration of 2.5% for a hazardous material that has a Permissible Exposure Limit (PEL) of 250 ppm and an Immediately Dangerous to Life and Health (IDLH) of 2500 ppm and a Lower Explosive Limit (LEL) of 25,000 ppm. You have been assigned the task of respirator selection for entry into this atmosphere. Which of the following statements is the most correct?
    A) The instrument shows a reading more than the PEL and IDLH.
    B) The instrument shows a reading below the PEL, IDLH and LEL.
    C) The direct reading instrument indicates a concentration below the LEL but above the IDLH and PEL.
    D) The instrument shows a reading equal to the LEL, which is above the IDLH and PEL.

7). When taking noise measurements in a non-reverberant environment, instructions often call for placing the microphone in the workers hearing zone. Which of the following best describes the hearing zone?
    A) A area surrounding the body for a distance of 12 inches.
    B) A hemisphere 9-18 inches in radius and centered on the shoulder.
    C) A hemisphere 6-9 inches in radius and forward of the shoulders.
    D) A sphere 2 ft in diameter centered on the head.

8). The primary health exposure concern with removal of old paint is
    A) Asbestos.
    B) Cadmium.
    C) Lead.
    D) Mercury.

9). Asbestos work includes repair and maintenance operations where ACM or presumed ACM (PACM) are disturbed is classified as
    A) Class I.
    B) Class II.
    C) Class III.
    D) Class IV.

10). A new addition will be added on to an existing building and workers have expressed a concern about asbestos exposure. The CHST should:
    A) Require respirators to be worn.
    B) Conduct asbestos awareness training.
    C) Verify that there is asbestos containing materials.
    D) Implement engineering controls.

11). A standard combustible gas indicator reads in _____?
    A) percentage of LEL.
    B) tenths of LEL.
    C) percentage of LFL.
    D) directly in tenths or hundredths.

12). A worker wearing a harness with a six-foot lanyard attached at waist-height could be subject to a maximum of _____ feet free fall?
    A) 6 feet.
    B) 8 feet.
    C) 3 feet.
    D) 9 feet.

13). In which of the following conditions would the use of dilution ventilation be most appropriate?
    A) The source is very toxic.
    B) The source of contamination is a heavy particulate.
    C) Employees are in close contact with the source.
    D) The source of contamination is constant.

14). All the following are recognized classes of protective footwear except?
  A) Conductive shoes/boots.
  B) Electrical Hazard Shoes/boots.
  C) Safety-Toe Safety Shoes Class "75".
  D) Non-ionizing, worker Safety Shoe Class "EX" radiation.

15). _____ is based on the rate of heat loss from exposed skin caused by wind and cold.
  A) Work temperature.
  B) Wind chill.
  C) Heat loss factor.
  D) Radiation decay.

16). You are on a safety survey of one of your work sites and discover a bulldozer is operating with its back up signal inoperable, you should?
  A) Have it fixed at the end of the work shift.
  B) Cease operations until it is fixed.
  C) Continue working with a qualified employee as a backup spotter.
  D) Continue working, ensuring the operator always clears behind the bulldozer before backing up.

17). Chemical labeling is best communicated in:
  A) English only.
  B) All languages present on the job site.
  C) A language that both management and workers understand.
  D) A language that workers understand.

18). Guardrails and toe boards are required for any construction scaffolding platform over _____ above the ground.
  A) 5 feet.
  B) 8 feet.
  C) 10 feet.
  D) 12 feet.

19). According to 29 CFR 1910.23, a standard railing shall consist of top rail, intermediate rail, and posts, and shall have a vertical height of ___ inches nominal from upper surface of top rail to floor, platform, runway, or ramp level.
  A) 36 inches.
  B) 40 inches.
  C) 42 inches.
  D) 48 inches.

20). When making a periodic inspection of chains, you should inspect the chain link-by-link, looking for all the following except?
  A) Bent links.
  B) Painted links.
  C) Corrosion pits.
  D) Stretching caused by overloading.

21). Which of the following would not require a label under the provisions of OSHA 1926.59, Hazard Communication standard?
  A) Fuel tank in a pickup truck at construction site.
  B) A storage tank of hazardous chemicals.
  C) A small container used to dispense chemicals by workers at the jobsite.
  D) Compressed gas cylinders.

22). The best method to splice a 0.5-inch wire rope is to:
  A) Create and eyelet, secure 3 clips with saddle on the live end.
  B) Create a knot, secure with 2 clips with saddle on the dead end.
  C) Create an eyelet, secure with 2 clips, with saddle on the live end.
  D) Create an eyelet, secure 2 clips with saddle on live end and one clip saddle on the dead end.

23). All the following substances are excluded from the OSHA Hazard Communication Standard labeling requirements except?
  A) Wood products including wood dust.
  B) Hazardous Waste.
  C) Alcoholic beverages.
  D) Pesticides.

24). Thoracic Outlet Syndrome is a disease caused by:
    A) An inflammation of a tendon.
    B) Compression of the ulnar nerve.
    C) Compression of the median nerve.
    D) Compression of nerves and blood vessels between clavicle and first and second ribs.

25). Safety nets requirements include:
    A) Not less than 8" x 8" netting.
    B) Extend 3 feet beyond the edge of working area.
    C) Extend 8 feet beyond the edge of working area.
    D) Nets must be positioned more than 30 feet below such work surface.

Domain 1: Quiz 4 Answers

1).   Answer C:

The MUC for respirators is calculated by multiplying the APF for the respirator by the PEL. The MUC is the upper limit at which the class of respirator is expected to provide protection.
The Protection Factor for a half-mask respirator from the chart is 10.

MUC = TLV x APF
$$= 10 \text{ mg/m}^3 \times 10$$
$$= 100 \text{ mg/m}^3$$

End-of-service-life indicator (ESLI) means a system that warns the respirator user of the approach of the end of adequate respiratory protection, for example, that the sorbent is approaching saturation or is no longer

2).   Answer C:

Both Ultraviolet (UV) and Infrared radiation (IR) will cause damage to the eye. However, IR is very penetrating and passes through the cornea to the retina of the eye causing permanent damage. Ultraviolet radiation will cause eye burn (Arc Eye) that is painful and disabling but usually the signs and symptoms disappear in 12 to 36 hours and, as stated earlier, confined to the cornea.

3).   Answer C:

Helmet Types
Class E (Electrical) helmets intended to reduce the danger of exposure to high voltage electrical conductors, proof tested at 20,000 volts. Class E is tested for force transmission first, then tested at 20,000 volts for 3 minutes, with 9 milliamps maximum current leakage; then tested at 30,000 volts, with no burn-through permitted. (formerly Class B)
Class G (General) helmets intended to reduce the danger of exposure to low voltage electrical conductors, proof tested at 2,200 volts. Class G is tested at 2,200 volts for 1 minute, with 3 milliamps max. leakage. (formerly Class A)
Class C (Conductive) helmets not intended to provide protection from electrical conductors. Class C is not tested for electrical resistance. (no change in class designation)

Definitions expanded; new test protocol section, including preparation, mounting, number, and sequence of test samples; summary of failure criteria.

- Product tested within 3-inch circle on top of helmet in "as worn" position
- 2.2-pound pointed steel penetrator, with 60° angle, dropped from a simulated free-fall height of 8 feet
- Penetrator can't make contact w/ head form
- Test apparatus includes electronic contact indicator, velocity indicator, & electronic recording equipment
- No differentiation for helmet classes

4).   Answer D:

Most of the energy is present above 1,000 cps. If there was a substantially lower reading on the "A" scale compared to the "C" scale an assumption could be made that most of the noise frequency was below 1,000 cps (due to the severe weighting of the "A" scale). However, in this case the readings are approximately the same, that indicates the noise must be in range where the two scales are not weighted significantly different.

Comparison of Sound Level Meter Scales

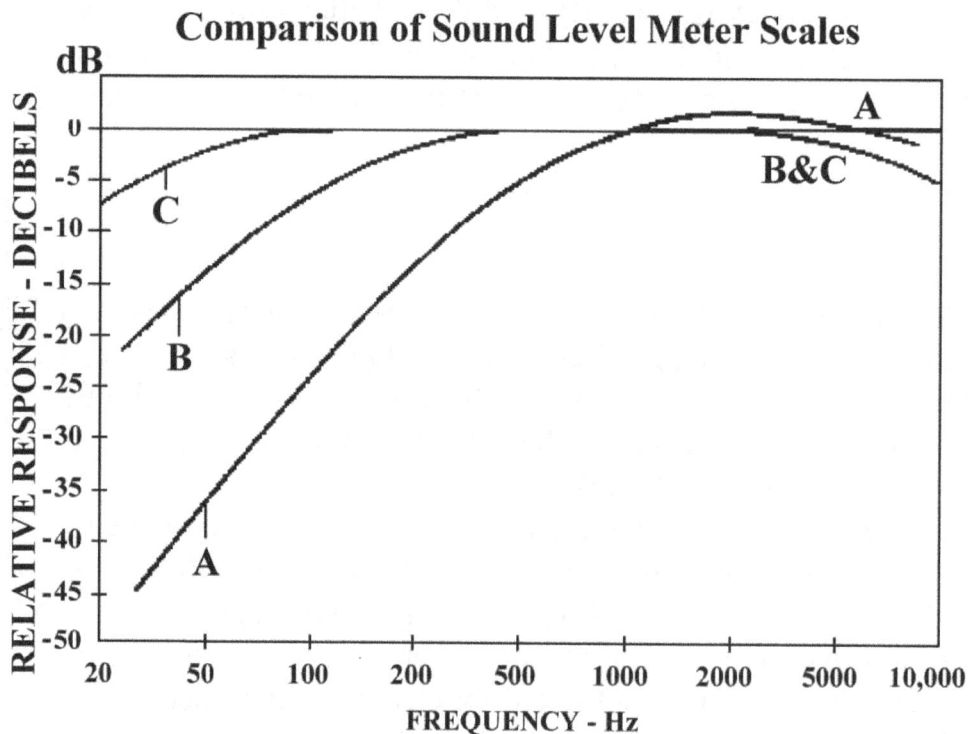

5). Answer C:

Overhead cranes can be equipped with a limit switch system to prevent the over travel of the load block. This attachment often referred to as a anti-two block device prevents the load block from being drawn into the sheeve or drum. In the illustration shown here a switch is attached to the crane boom. The switch is held in the closed position by a weight that slides down the hoisting line. When the load block comes too close to the point sheave the weight is lifted and allows the spring-loaded switch to open and disconnect power to the hoist apparatus.

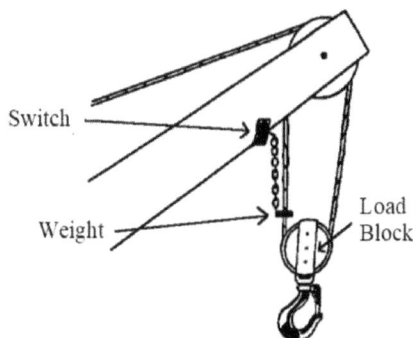

Anti-two-block damage prevention system
OSHA 1926.550

6). Answer D:

$$ppm = \% \times 1,000,000$$
$$ppm = 2.5\% \times 1,000,000$$
$$ppm = 25,000$$

Convert percent to ppm and compare to LEL. From the comparison the concentration is above both the PEL and the IDLH but equal to the LEL.
PELs- OSHA Permissible Exposure Limits are time weighted average (TWA) concentrations that must not be exceeded during any 8-hour work shift of a 40-hour workweek.
IDLHs- By NIOSH definition Immediately dangerous to life or health concentrations represent the maximum concentration from which, in the event of respirator failure, one could escape within 30 minutes without a respirator and without experiencing any escape-impairing (e.g., severe eye irritation) or irreversible health effects.

LEL-UEL- Lower Explosive Limit or Lower Flammable Limit. By NFPA definition lower flammable limit is the minimum concentration of vapor to air below which propagation of a flame will not occur in the presence of an ignition source. The UEL or upper flammable limit is the maximum vapor-to-air concentration above which propagation of flame will not occur. At or below the UEL it can ignite. The area bounded by the LEL and the UEL is called the flammability range.

7). Answer D:

The general agreement within the safety and health community concerning placement of a sound recording instrument microphone is the closer to the workers ear the better. However, the agreed upon definition of hearing zone is a sphere with a two-foot diameter surrounding the head. Selection "C" is the preferred definition of Breathing Zone.

8). Answer C:

OSHA 29 CFR 1926.62 is the standard for Lead in Construction. Employees in the construction industry may be exposed to lead in several forms:
- Lead itself is used on some electrical and elevator cables and on cast-iron soil pipe installation.
- Removing old lead paint and rust from bridges and other industrial structures.
- Renovating, remodeling, or repainting pre 1978 houses and buildings.
- Lead remediation.
- Lead solder is used in some industrial construction.
- Lead-containing mortar is used in some tanks.
- Pure lead and lead products, including lead panels (drywall/plywood), lead bricks, and lead shot, are used for shielding numerous military, industrial, research, and medical radiation sources.
- Stained-glass windows may contain lead.
- Lead use as a component in paint.

9).   Answer C:

The OSHA standard establishes a classification system for asbestos construction work that spells out mandatory, simple, technological work practices that employers must follow to reduce worker exposures. Under this system, the following four classes of construction work are matched with increasingly stringent control requirements:

- *Class I* asbestos work is the most potentially hazardous class of asbestos jobs. This work involves the removal of asbestos-containing thermal system insulation and sprayed-on or troweled-on surfacing materials. Employers must presume that thermal system insulation and surfacing material found in pre-1981 construction is ACM. That presumption, however, is rebuttable. If you believe that the surfacing material or thermal system insulation is not ACM, the OSHA standard specifies the means that you must use to rebut that presumption. Thermal system insulation includes ACM applied to pipes, boilers, tanks, ducts, or other structural components to prevent heat loss or gain. Surfacing materials include decorative plaster on ceilings and walls; acoustical materials on decking, walls, and ceilings; and fireproofing on structural members.
- *Class II* work includes the removal of other types of ACM that are not thermal system insulation such as resilient flooring and roofing materials. Examples of Class II work include removal of asbestos-containing floor or ceiling tiles, siding, roofing, or transite panels.
- *Class III* asbestos work includes repair and maintenance operations where ACM or presumed ACM (PACM) are disturbed.
- *Class IV* work includes custodial activities where employees clean up asbestos-containing waste and debris produced by construction, maintenance, or repair activities. This work involves cleaning dust-contaminated surfaces, vacuuming contaminated carpets, mopping floors, and cleaning up ACM or PACM from thermal system insulation or surfacing material.

10). Answer C:

Employers discovering ACM on a worksite must notify the building/facility owner and other employers onsite within 24 hours regarding its presence, location, and quantity. You also must inform owners and employees working in nearby areas of the precautions taken to confine airborne asbestos. Within 10 days of project completion, you must inform building/facility owners and other employers onsite of the current locations and quantities of remaining ACM and any final monitoring results. At any time, employers or building and facility owners may demonstrate that a PACM does not contain asbestos by inspecting the material in accordance with the requirements of the *Asbestos Hazard Emergency Response Act* (AHERA) (40 CFR Part 763, Subpart E) or by performing tests of bulk samples collected in the manner described in 40 CFR Part 763.86. (See 29 CFR Part 1926.1101 for specific testing requirements.) Employers do not have to inform employees of asbestos free building materials present; however, you must retain the information, data, and analysis supporting the determination.

11) Answer A:

The standard hot wire combustible gas detector reads in percent LEL. The most important factor for maximizing the reliability of direct-reading electrical and electronic instruments is to calibrate when recommend by the technical orders.

12) Answer A:

For a belt and 6-foot lanyard a waist-height attachment would produce a 6-foot free fall. **1926.502(d)(15)** Anchorages used for attachment of personal fall arrest equipment shall be independent of any anchorage being used to support or suspend platforms and capable of supporting at least 5,000 pounds (22.2 kN) per employee attached, or shall be designed, installed, and used as follows: as part of a complete personal fall arrest system which maintains a safety factor of at least two; and under the supervision of a qualified person.
1926.502(d)(16) Personal fall arrest systems, when stopping a fall, shall:
- limit maximum arresting force on an employee to 900 pounds (4 kN) when used with a body belt;
- limit maximum arresting force on an employee to 1,800 pounds (8 kN) when used with a body harness;
- be rigged such that an employee can neither free fall more than 6 feet

(1.8 m), nor contact any lower level;

- bring an employee to a complete stop and limit maximum deceleration distance an employee travels to 3.5 feet (1.07 m); and,
- have sufficient strength to withstand twice the potential impact energy of an employee free falling a distance of 6 feet (1.8 m), or the free fall distance permitted by the system, whichever is less.

1926.502(d)(19) Personal fall arrest systems and components subjected to impact loading shall be immediately removed from service and shall not be used again for employee protection until inspected and determined by a competent person to be undamaged and suitable for reuse.

1926.502(e) "Positioning device systems.": Positioning device systems and their use shall conform to the following provisions: Positioning devices shall be rigged such that an employee cannot free fall more than 2 feet (.9 m). Positioning devices shall be secured to an anchorage capable of supporting at least twice the potential impact load of an employee's fall or 3,000 pounds (13.3 kN), whichever is greater.

13) Answer D:

Dilution ventilation is the preferred solution when relatively non-toxic emissions are produced, when the source is mainly gases or vapors (not primarily heavy particulates) and when employees do not work in the immediate vicinity or direct path of the emission source. The old adage "no pollution through more dilution" is often very appropriate, however when toxic, heavy, direct path, time inconsistent, or large sources of emissions are encountered the solution is point source removal through local exhaust ventilation.

14) Answer D:

There is not a category of protective footwear designed especially for Non-ionizing radiation workers. *Conductive footwear* offering a resistance below 450k OHMs is available to allow for dissipation of static charges. Typical applications would include some types of munitions manufacturing, cleaning tanks that have contained flammable liquids, etc. The *ANSI Std. Z41 "Safety-Toe Footwear"* groups Safety Toe Footwear into three classes which indicates the impact weight the shoes are designed to withstand while maintaining a

16/32 (15/32 for women) inch clearance inside the shoe. The classes are 75, 50 and 30. Electrical hazard shoes are designed to lessen the hazards of contact with electrical current. There are various special types of protective footwear that have extra protection from protruding nails, hot surfaces etc.

15)   Answer B:

The wind chill temperature is how cold people and animals feel when outside. Wind chill is based on the rate of heat loss from exposed skin caused by wind and cold. As the wind increases, it draws heat from the body, driving down skin temperature and eventually the internal body temperature. Therefore, the wind makes it FEEL much colder. If the temperature is 0 degrees Fahrenheit and the wind is blowing at 15 mph, the wind chill is -19 degrees Fahrenheit. At this wind chill temperature, exposed skin can freeze in 30 minutes. Wind Chill Factor is caused by increased wind speeds which accelerate heat loss from exposed skin. No specific rules exist for determining when wind chill becomes dangerous. As a general rule, the threshold for potentially dangerous wind chill conditions is about -20°F. Wind chill factor is the major concern when exposing workers to the elements.

16)   Answer C:

This is a difficult question because many places in the standard it states the warning device must be operable, however there is an exception that allows operation when "an employee signals that it is safe to do so".
1926.602(a)(9)(i): All bidirectional machines, such as rollers, compacters, front-end loaders, bulldozers, and similar equipment, shall be equipped with a horn, distinguishable from the surrounding noise level, which shall be operated as needed when the machine is moving in either direction. The horn shall be maintained in an operative condition.
1926.602(a)(9)(ii): No employer shall permit earthmoving or compacting equipment which has an obstructed view to the rear to be used in reverse gear unless the equipment has in operation a reverse signal alarm distinguishable from the surrounding noise level or an employee signals that it is safe to do so.

17)   Answer C:

The Globally Harmonized System (GHS) of classification and labeling of chemicals provides a standardized approach, including detailed criteria for determining what hazardous effects a chemical presents, as well as standardized label elements assigned by hazard class and category. This will enhance both employer and worker comprehension of the hazards, which will help to ensure appropriate handling and safe use of workplace chemicals. In addition, the safety data sheet requirements establish an order of information that is standardized. The harmonized format of the safety data sheets will enable employers, workers, health professionals, and emergency responders to access the information more efficiently and effectively, thus increasing their utility.

18)   Answer C:

With few exceptions, guardrails and toeboards are required on platforms over 10 feet above the ground. OSHA (1926.451) CAUTION: The general industry standards at 1910.23 generally require a standard guardrail anytime a drop of more than 4 feet is encountered.

19)   Answer C:

29 CFR 1910.23(e)(1): A standard railing shall consist of top rail, intermediate rail, and posts, and shall have a vertical height of 42 inches nominal from upper surface of top rail to floor, platform, runway, or ramp level. The top rail shall be smooth-surfaced throughout the length of the railing. The intermediate rail shall be approximately halfway between the top rail and the floor, platform, runway, or ramp. The ends of the rails shall not overhang the terminal posts except where such overhang does not constitute a projection hazard.
29 CFR 1910.23(e)(4): A standard toeboard shall be 4 inches nominal in vertical height from its top edge to the level of the floor, platform, runway, or ramp. It shall be securely fastened in place and with not more than 1/4-inch clearance above floor level. It may be made of any substantial material either solid or with openings not over 1 inch in greatest dimension.

20) Answer B:

According to the National Safety Council, a link-by-link inspection should be made to detect the following:

- bent links
- cracks in weld areas, in shoulders or in any other section of link
- transverse nicks or gouges
- corrosion pits
- stretching caused by overloading

21) Answer A:

Labels are required on all of the items listed in the question except the fuel tank on the pickup truck, which is exempt.
1910.1200(f)(5) Except as provided in paragraphs (f)(6) and (f)(7) of this section, the employer shall ensure that each container of hazardous chemicals in the workplace is labeled, tagged or marked with the following information: identity of the hazardous chemical(s) contained therein; and, appropriate hazard warnings, or alternatively, words, pictures, symbols, or combination thereof, which provide at least general information regarding the hazards of the chemicals, and which, in conjunction with the other information immediately available to employees under the hazard communication program, will provide employees with the specific information regarding the physical and health hazards of the hazardous chemical.

22) Answer A:

OSHA 29 CFR 1926.251 states that for a half inch wire rope, when U-bolt wire rope clips are used to form eyes, there must be 3 clips, saddles on the live end. Wire rope shall not be used if, in any length of eight diameters, the total number of visible broken wires exceeds 10 percent of the total number of wires, or if the rope shows other signs of excessive wear, corrosion, or defect.

23)   Answer A:

The OSHA Hazard Communication Standard does not cover some materials that come under regulation by government agencies other than OSHA. Included are alcohol, hazardous waste, pesticides and wood products. However, the exemption does not include wood dust and the OSHA PEL for wood dust must be included in the SDS for such products. Additionally, any wood additives present in the wood, which represent a health hazard, must also be included on the SDSs or label.

24)   Answer D:

Thoracic outlet syndrome is defined as a disorder resulting from a compression of nerves and blood vessels between clavicle and first and second ribs at the brachial plexus. Can be caused by typing, keying, carrying heavy loads or keeping the head, arms and/or shoulders in an unnatural position.

25)   Answer C:

According to 1926.105, Safety nets shall be provided when workplaces are more than 25 feet above the ground or water surface, or other surfaces where the use of ladders, scaffolds, catch platforms, temporary floors, safety lines, or safety belts is impractical. Nets shall extend 8 feet beyond the edge of the work surface where employees are exposed and shall be installed as close under the work surface as practical but in no case more than 25 feet below such work surface. Nets shall be hung with sufficient clearance to prevent user's contact with the surfaces or structures below. Such clearances shall be determined by impact load testing. The mesh size of nets shall not exceed 6 inches by 6 inches. All new nets shall meet accepted performance standards of 17,500 foot-pounds minimum impact resistance as determined and certified by the manufacturers and shall bear a label of proof test. Edge ropes shall provide a minimum breaking strength of 5,000 pounds.

Domain 1: Quiz 5 Questions

1). One of the critical operations during the lift is keeping the slab level, and is often automatically controlled. How much tolerance is permitted between lifting points when jacking the slab?

A) Two feet.
B) One inch.
C) Six inches.
D) ½ inch.

2). Transfer of weight from the jacks to the building support columns cannot take place until the welds on the shear plates have achieved maximum strength. Accordingly, the weight cannot be transferred until?

A) The welds have cooled for 30 minutes.
B) The welds have cooled for 5 minutes.
C) The welds have cooled to 120 degrees.
D) The welds have cooled to air temperature.

3). All the following requirements for concrete mixers or tools are true **except**?

A) Tremies must have wire rope safeties in addition to couplings.
B) Concrete buckets with hydraulic gates must have safety latches.
C) Power trowels are not required to be equipped with dead man switches.
D) Concrete pumping system air hoses must have fail-safe connectors.

4). Which of the following is true concerning electrically operated hand-held power tools on the construction site?

A) All power tools must be grounded.
B) Double insulated tools do not need to be grounded.
C) Power operated tools must be connected to a GFCI when used outdoors.
D) GFCIs are required on construction sites.

5). During a training session on hazardous material labeling, you are referring to the NFPA 704, Identification of Hazards of Materials. During this presentation you should properly identify what color and purpose for the left diamond?

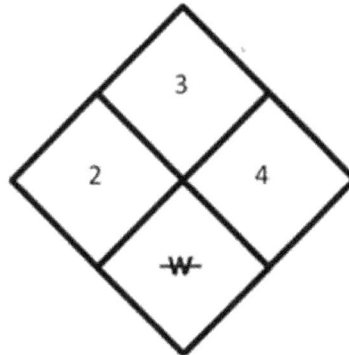

    A) Blue, fire.
    B) Yellow, fire.
    C) Red, fire.
    D) Blue, health.

6). During a training session it is stated that the pH is a measure of a materials acidity or alkalinity. What would a pH of 2 indicate?
    A) A very strong acid.
    B) A basic mixture used for building other compounds.
    C) An alkaline.
    D) A mixture of compounds.

7). A safety orientation session might include the information that the A-weighted sound level measurement is used as the "standard" scale in occupational noise measurement:
    A) It weights intermittent and impact noise.
    B) Weighing is related to effects of noise on the ear.
    C) It filters out "white" noise.
    D) It has a built-in dose response curve.

8). When required to use PPE, the employee must be training in all the areas except?
    A) How to purchase PPE.
    B) When PPE is necessary.
    C) The limitations of the PPE.
    D) How to properly don, doff, adjust, and wear PPE.

9). Ladder jack scaffolds platforms **shall not** exceed a height of ___ ?
   A) 10 feet.
   B) 20 feet.
   C) 25 feet.
   D) 30 feet.

10). Hazardous chemical labels should be written in:
   A) In a language and symbols that workers can read and identify hazards.
   B) English only.
   C) English and Spanish.
   D) According to North American or European standards.

11). The **best** solution to a hazard on the jobsite is:
   A) Barricade the hazard.
   B) Eliminate the hazard.
   C) Train affected workers on hazard.
   D) Continue work and report hazard to controlling employer.

12). The 4 in the diagram indicates:

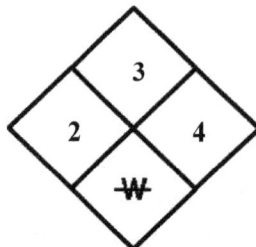

   A) Health.
   B) Fire.
   C) Reactivity.
   D) Storage.

13). What is the maximum height steel erection workers may free climb without fall protection?
   A) 6 feet.
   B) 15 feet.
   C) 12 feet.
   D) 10 feet.

14). Which of the following best describes the Threshold Limit Value?
   A) The amount of hazardous chemical exposure to which a worker can be exposed.
   B) The number of physical hazards to which a worker can be exposed.
   C) The amount of hazardous chemicals in work area.
   D) The required information on a container label.

15). If an employee owns her own PPE, who is responsible to ensure it is maintained?
   A) Employee.
   B) Employer.
   C) Union Rep.
   D) Supervisor.

16). What does the illustrated crane hand signals indicate?
   A) All stop / emergency stop.
   B) Move slowly.
   C) Use auxiliary hoist.
   D) Stop.

17). What is the safety factor on wire ropes for Suspended Scaffolding?
   A) 2:1
   B) 4:1
   C) 6:1
   D) 8:1

18). An example of an acute exposure is:
   A) Lung cancer.
   B) Dizziness from a sudden drop in blood pressure.
   C) Mesothelioma.
   D) Meniere's disease.

19). Which of these would be above the exposure limit?
   A) 92 dBA for 8 hours.
   B) 105 dBA for 45 minutes.
   C) 110 dBA for 20 minutes.
   D) 115 dBA for 10 minutes.

20). For electrical safety on construction sites, OSHA requires employers to ensure either GFCIs or:
    A) UL certified extension cords.
    B) A scheduled and recorded assured equipment grounding conductor program.
    C) That all electrical tools have grounding (3-prong) plugs.
    D) That all electrical tools are double insulated.

21). Fixed ladders must have side rails that extend at least how far above the top landing surface?
    A) 24 inches.
    B) 36 inches.
    C) 42 inches.
    D) 44 inches.

22). Once you have left a confined space, what actions would you need to take to re-enter that space?
    A) Fill out an entirely new permit and submit it for approval.
    B) Call OSHA and file a formal complaint.
    C) File a photo copy of the previous permit considering the space is likely the same.
    D) Verify that appropriate controls have been implemented and that all conditions are safe for re-entry.

23). What is the **best** way to prevent trench cave-ins?
    A) Sloping.
    B) Covering.
    C) Placing spoil piles away from edge of trench.
    D) Shoring.

24). How many wires may be damaged in one strand a wire rope sling rope lay before the sling is taken out of service?
    A) One wire in one strand of a rope lay.
    B) Two wires in one strand of a rope lay.
    C) Five wires in one strand of a rope lay.
    D) No wires can be cut in one strand of a rope lay.

25). In what order do you test the atmosphere in a confined space?

    A) Oxygen, Flammability, Toxicity.

    B) Flammability, Oxygen, Toxicity.

    C) Toxicity, Flammability, Oxygen.

    D) Order of testing is irrelevant.

Domain 1: Quiz 5 Answers

1)   Answer D:

The requirements for lift-slab operations are very stringent and operations receive a lot of attention from OSHA because of the potential for large accidental loss. All lift-slab operations must be designed and planned by a registered professional engineer (P.E.). Jacks and lifting devices must be capable of supporting at least 2½ times the load to be lifted and cannot be overloaded.
Only ½ inch tolerance is permitted between jacking points when raising the slab during lift-slab operations. Generally this operation is done automatically, however it is permissible to maintain the leveling manually when the lifting controls are centrally located and there are no more than 14 jacks.

2)   Answer D:

The requirements for lift-slab operations are very stringent and operations receive a lot of attention from OSHA because of the potential for large accidental loss. All lift-slab operations must be designed and planned by a registered professional engineer (P.E.). After the slab is lifted into position by jacks/lifting units, the slab can be positively secured to the building columns. All welding must be done by certified welders, familiar with the plans and specifications for the lift-slab operation.

To ensure maximum strength has developed in any welded surface, the load transfer from the jacks/lifting units to the building columns, during lift-slab operations, cannot take place until welds on the column shear plates or weld blocks are cooled to air temperature.

3)   Answer C:

Selection "A" is true, tremies, or elephant trunks, are tubes connected to a hopper and are used to place concrete. They are used extensively for under water placement. If the coupling fails on a tremie, workers could obviously be hurt, so they must be secured by an extra method, most often wire rope is used as an attachment. Selection "B" is also true, concrete buckets with power gates or valves must have positive latches to prevent dumping material should the power source fail, eg: loss of hydraulic or air pressure. Selection "D" is also correct, OSHA requires positive fail-safe joint connectors on concrete pumping system compressed air hoses. This is to prevent accidental separation of the hose sections while they are pressurized. Selection "C" is of course false, power concrete trowels must be equipped with a dead man switch that shuts down the power to the trowel if the operator should let go of the handle. Power trowels are very powerful, if the trigger is bypassed or taped down and the trowel gets loose, it can cause several anxious moments on the construction site.

4)   Answer B:

Double insulated tools do not require equipment grounding due to the extra protection provided by the insulation. Selection "A" is not true, tools that are double or triple insulated do not have to be grounded. Key word here is "ALL". Selection "C" is not true, power operated tools could be used outdoors if the site had an assured grounding program. Selection "D" is not true, GFCIs are not required on construction sites, the alternative is an assured grounding program.

5)   Answer D:

NFPA 704

Health
4. Extreme danger
3. Great danger
2. Hazardous
1. Irritating
0. Ordinary

W—
OX

Flammability
4. Extremely flammable
3. Ignition at normal temperatures.
2. Ignition when moderately heated
1. Must be preheated to
0. Noncombustible

Reactivity
4. May detonate
3. Strong shock or heat may
2. Violent chemical reaction possible
1. Unstable if heated
0. Normally stable

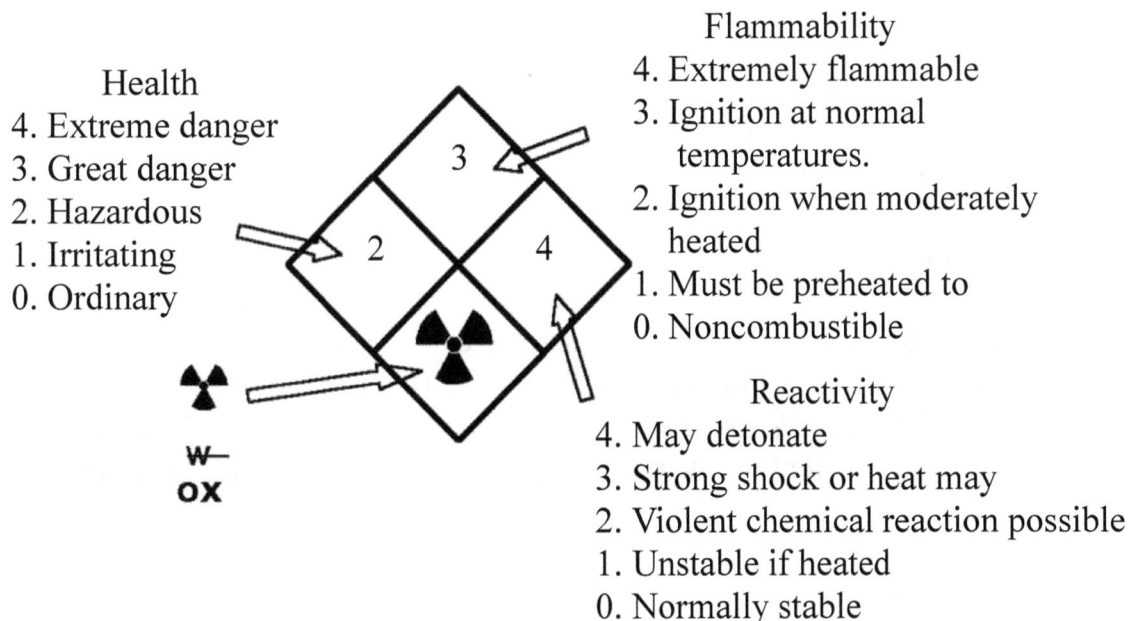

According to the National Fire Protection Association Handbook, the NFPA 704, Identification of the Hazards of Materials is a symbol system intended for use on fixed installations or buildings. It tells the fire fighters what they must do to protect themselves. The system is based on the NFPA Standard 704 diamond that visually presents information on health, flammability, and the self-reactivity hazard of a material. NFPA 704 describes in great detail the hazards and hazard level which the various numbers indicate for the three hazards. Numbers from 0 through 4 are placed in the three upper diamonds to show the degree of hazard present. The 0 indicates the lowest degree of hazard, 4 indicates the highest. The five categories of *health* hazards are presented in the left diamond, which is colored blue. *Fire* hazards are presented in the top diamond, which is colored red. *Reactivity* (stability) hazards are presented in the right diamond, which is colored yellow. Additionally, special information is presented in the bottom diamond, which is colored white, to convey the dangers of high-risk materials.

The five degrees of hazard shown above have the following general meaning to fire fighters:

4	Too dangerous to approach with standard fire fighting equipment and procedures. Withdraw and obtain expert advice on how to handle.
3	Fire can be fought using methods intended for extremely hazardous situations, such as unmanned monitors or personal protective equipment, which prevents all bodily contact.
2	Can be fought with standard procedures, but hazards are present which require certain equipment or procedures to handle safety.
1	Nuisance hazards present, which require some care, but standard fire fighting procedures can be used.
0	No special hazards, therefore no special measures.

6) Answer A:

The pH is a number that indicates the acidity or alkalinity of an aqueous solution. The range of the pH scale is from 0 to 14. Aqueous solutions having a pH from 0 to 7 are *acidic*. Aqueous solutions having a pH from 7 to 14 are basic, or caustic, or alkaline. A material having a pH of 2 would be a very strong acid.

7) Answer B:

The A-weighted scale most closely weights the sound to the injurious effects of the noise on the ear.

8) Answer A:

1910.132(f)(1)
The employer shall provide training to each employee who is required by this section to use PPE. Each such employee shall be trained to know at least the following:

- When PPE is necessary;
- What PPE is necessary;
- How to properly don, doff, adjust, and wear PPE;
- The limitations of the PPE; and,
- The proper care, maintenance, useful life and disposal of the PPE.

1910.132(f)(2)
Each affected employee shall demonstrate an understanding of the training specified in paragraph (f)(1) of this section, and the ability to use PPE properly, before being allowed to perform work requiring the use of PPE.

9) Answer B:

1926.452(k) - "Ladder jack scaffolds." Platforms shall not exceed a height of 20 feet (6.1 m).

All ladders used to support ladder jack scaffolds shall meet the requirements of subpart X of this part -- Stairways and Ladders, except that job-made ladders shall not be used to support ladder jack scaffolds.

The ladder jack shall be so designed and constructed that it will bear on the side rails and ladder rungs or on the ladder rungs alone. If bearing on rungs only, the bearing area shall include a length of at least 10 inches (25.4 cm) on each rung.

10) Answer A:

Hazardous chemical labels should be written in a language and symbols so that workers can read and identify hazard

11)   Answer B:

Training is not always the best solution to a safety issue. Hazard elimination is the best solution although the process of elimination may present new substitution hazards that require employee training.

Safety management requires following the hierarchies of control.
  1)   Engineering,
  2)   Administrative (Training),
  3)   PPE

12)   Answer C:

The NFPA 704 System Hazard Diamond is a symbol system intended for use of

NFPA 704 Symbol

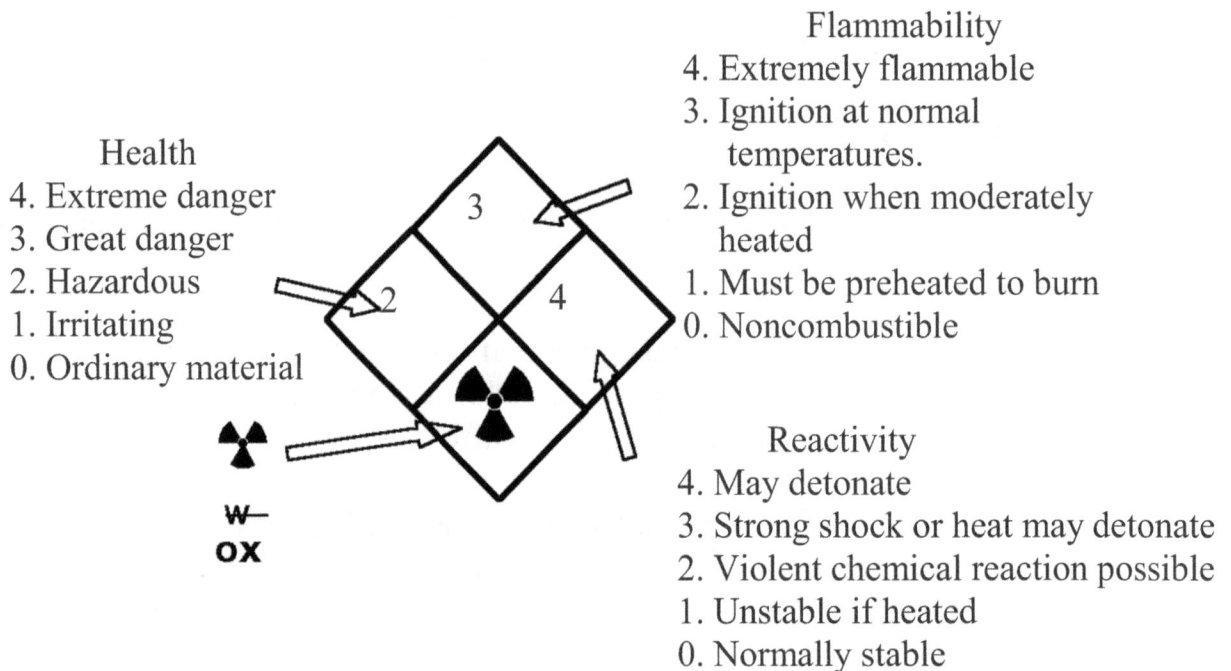

Health
4. Extreme danger
3. Great danger
2. Hazardous
1. Irritating
0. Ordinary material

Flammability
4. Extremely flammable
3. Ignition at normal
   temperatures.
2. Ignition when moderately
   heated
1. Must be preheated to burn
0. Noncombustible

Reactivity
4. May detonate
3. Strong shock or heat may detonate
2. Violent chemical reaction possible
1. Unstable if heated
0. Normally stable

W—
OX

fixed installations, such as chemical processing equipment, storage and warehousing rooms and laboratory entrances. It tells a fire fighter what he must do to protect himself from injury while fighting a fire in the area. In this diamond, the four is the reactivity diamond.

13)   Answer B:

In steel erection, a new, very narrow working surface is constantly being created as skeletal steel is erected at various heights. For many steel erectors, especially connectors, the work starts at the top level of the structure. This means that anchor points above foot level are often limited or unavailable. The special circumstances of steel erection can make conventional fall protection very difficult to deploy below 15 feet. For this reason, the following requirements and exceptions in the the steel erection fall protection standard have been made. [29 CFR 1926.760]

- Employees who are on a walking/working surface with an unprotected edge more than *15 feet above a lower level* must be protected by conventional fall protection.
- *Perimeter safety cables* must be installed at the final interior and exterior perimeters of multi-story structures *as soon as the decking has been installed.*
- Connectors and employees working in *controlled decking zones* must be protected from fall hazards.
- Connectors must be protected by *conventional fall protection* when working on a surface with an unprotected edge *more than two stories or 30 feet* above a lower level. Workers must have completed the *connector training*
- While working at heights *over 15 and up to 30 feet*, connectors must:
  - ○ Be provided with a complete *personal fall arrest system* or other allowable fall protection.
  - ○ *Wear the equipment* necessary for tying off.
- A CDZ can be established as a substitute for fall protection where metal decking is initially being installed and forms the *leading edge* of a work area *over 15 and up to 30 feet* above a lower level.
- Leading-edge workers in a CDZ are required to:
- Be protected from fall hazards *above 2 stories or 30 feet (whichever is less)*.
  - ○ Have *completed CDZ training*
  - ○ Employees who are not engaged in leading-edge work and properly trained in the hazards involved are *prohibited from entering* the CDZ.
- The CDZ is required to:
  - ○ Be no more than *90 feet wide and 90 feet deep* from any leading edge.

- o Not exceed *3,000 square feet* of unsecured decking. Have designated and clearly marked *boundaries with control lines* or the equivalent. *NOTE:* Control lines are commonly used as a marker because they create a highly visible boundary.
- o Have *safety deck attachments* placed from the leading edge back to the control line.
- o Have at least *two safety deck attachments* for each metal decking panel.
- o *Final deck attachments* and the installation of *shear connectors* are prohibited from being done in the CDZ.

The steel erector may *leave fall protection in place* so it may be used by other trades only if the *controlling contractor*:

- o Has *directed the steel erector* to leave the fall protection in place.
- o Has *inspected and accepted control and responsibility* of the fall protection before authorizing other trades to work in the area.

14)   Answer A:

The TLV lists the exposure amount for chemicals and is published by the American Conference of Government Industrial Hygienists (ACGIH).

15)   Answer B:

1910.132(b) Employee-owned equipment: Where employees provide their own protective equipment, the employer shall be responsible to assure its adequacy, including proper maintenance, and sanitation of such equipment.

16)   Answer A:

Swinging both arms back and forth while they are extended horizontally with palms down is the signal for emergency stop. Learn all the hand and arm signals from Appendix A to Subpart CC of Part 1926--Standard Hand Signals, shown here:

LOWER THE BOOM AND RAISE THE LOAD – With arm extended horizontally to the side and thumb pointing down, fingers open and close while load movement is desired.	**MOVE SLOWLY** – A hand is placed in front of the hand that is giving the action signal.	**USE AUXILIARY HOIST** (whipline) – With arm bent at elbow and forearm vertical, elbow is tapped with other hand. Then regular signal is used to indicate desired action.
CRAWLER CRANE TRAVEL, BOTH TRACKS – Rotate fists around each other in front of body; direction of rotation away from body indicates travel forward; rotation towards body indicates travel backward.	**USE MAIN HOIST** – A hand taps on top of the head. Then regular signal is given to indicate desired action.	**CRAWLER CRANE TRAVEL, ONE TRACK** – Indicate track to be locked by raising fist on that side. Rotate other fist in front of body in direction that other track is to travel.
TROLLEY TRAVEL – With palm up, fingers closed and thumb pointing in direction of motion, hand is jerked horizontally in direction trolley is to travel.		

STOP – With arm extended horizontally to the side, palm down, arm is swung back and forth.	**EMERGENCY STOP** – With both arms extended horizontally to the side, palms down, arms are swung back and forth.	**HOIST** – With upper arm extended to the side, forearm and index finger pointing straight up, hand and finger make small circles.
RAISE BOOM – With arm extended horizontally to the side, thumb points up with other fingers closed.	**SWING** – With arm extended horizontally, index finger points in direction that boom is to swing.	**RETRACT TELESCOPING BOOM** – With hands to the front at waist level, thumbs point at each other with other fingers closed.
RAISE THE BOOM AND LOWER THE LOAD – With arm extended horizontally to the side and thumb pointing up, fingers open and close while load movement is desired.	**DOG EVERYTHING** – Hands held together at waist level.	**LOWER** – With arm and index finger pointing down, hand and finger make small circles.
LOWER BOOM – With arm extended horizontally to the side, thumb points down with other fingers closed.	**EXTEND TELESCOPING BOOM** – With hands to the front at waist level, thumbs point outward with other fingers closed.	**TRAVEL/TOWER TRAVEL** – With all fingers pointing up, arm is extended horizontally out and back to make a pushing motion in the direction of travel.

17).   Answer C:

1926.451(a)(4) states "Each suspension rope, including connecting hardware, used on adjustable suspension scaffolds shall be capable of supporting, without failure, at least 6 times the maximum intended load applied or transmitted to that rope with the scaffold operating at either the rated load of the hoist, or 2 (minimum) times the stall load of the hoist, whichever is greater."

18). Answer B:

According to the Department of Health and Human Services, "Chemical exposures are generally divided into two categories: acute and chronic. Symptoms resulting from acute exposures usually occur during or shortly after exposure to a sufficiently high concentration of a contaminant." (Occupational Safety and Health Guidance Manual for Hazardous Waste Site Activities) Lung cancer, Mesothelioma and Meniere's disease all result from exposures over an extended period of time. Dizziness from a sudden drop in blood pressure could happen in just a few seconds or less.

19). Answer A:

1926.52(a) states "Protection against the effects of noise exposure shall be provided when the sound levels exceed those shown in Table D-2 of this section when **measured on the A-scale** of a standard sound level meter at slow response."
In all cases where the sound levels exceed the values shown herein, a continuing, effective hearing conservation program shall be administered. [1926.52(d)(1)]

TABLE D-2 - PERMISSIBLE NOISE EXPOSURES	
Duration per day, hours	Sound level dBA slow response
8	90
6	92
4	95
3	97
2	100
1 ½	102
1	105
½	110
1/4 or less	115

In addition, "If the variations in noise level involve **maxima at intervals of 1 second or less**, it is to be considered **continuous**." [1926.52(c)]

20).   Answer B:

OSHA states in Publication 3007: "Ground-fault protection rules and regulations have been determined necessary and appropriate for employee safety and health. Therefore, it is the employer's responsibility to provide either: (a) GFCIs on construction sites for receptacle outlets in use and not part of the permanent wiring of the building or structure; or (b) a scheduled and recorded assured equipment grounding conductor program on construction sites, covering all cord sets, receptacles which are not part of the permanent wiring of the building or structure, and equipment connected by cord and plug which are available for use or used by employees.

The employer is required to provide approved GFCIs for all 120-volt, single-phase, 15- and 20-ampere receptacle outlets on construction sites that are not a part of the permanent wiring of the building or structure and that are in use by employees. If a receptacle or receptacles are installed as part of the permanent wiring of the building or structure and they are used for temporary electric power, GFCI protection shall be provided. Receptacles on the ends of extension cords are not part of the permanent wiring and, therefore the cord's receptacle, must be of the GFCI type whether or not the extension cord is plugged into permanent wiring. These GFCIs monitor the current-to-the-load for leakage to ground."   *https://www.osha.gov/Publications/3007/3007.html*

21).   Answer C:

1926.1053(a)(24) states "The side rails of through or side-step fixed ladders shall extend 42 inches (1.1 m) above the top of the access level or landing platform served by the ladder. For a parapet ladder, the access level shall be the roof if the parapet is cut to permit passage through the parapet; if the parapet is continuous, the access level shall be the top of the parapet."

For portable ladders used to access an upper landing surface, the side rails must extend at least 3 feet (.9 m) above the upper landing surface.

22). Answer D:

Although you have already had individuals in the space that only had to leave due to a scheduling issue, some other emergency (not involving the conditions in the confined space), or any other issue, once you have left the space you must approach re-entry as if it is the initial entry. **All the entry requirements for testing and potential hazard identification apply equally to re-entry events just like initial entry**.

https://www.osha.gov/dte/grant_materials/fy09/sh-18796-09/confinedspace.pdf

23). Answer D:

OSHA states "There are different types of protective systems. Sloping involves cutting back the trench wall at an angle inclined away from the excavation. Shoring requires installing aluminum hydraulic or other types of supports to prevent soil movement and cave-ins. Shielding protects workers by using trench boxes or other types of supports to prevent soil cave-ins. Designing a protective system can be complex because you must consider many factors: soil classification, depth of cut, water content of soil, changes due to weather or climate, surcharge loads (eg., spoil, other materials to be used in the trench) and other operations in the vicinity." *https://www.osha.gov/Publications/trench_excavation_fs.html*

24). Answer C:

The OSHA Pub 3072, Sling Safety, states for *Wire Rope Sling Inspection* "Wire rope slings must be visually inspected before each day's use. The operator should check the twists or lay of the sling. If ten randomly distributed wires in one lay are broken, or **five wires in one strand of a rope lay are damaged**, the sling must not be used. It is not sufficient, however, to check only the condition of the wire rope. End fittings and other components should also be inspected for any damage that could make the sling unsafe." *https://www.osha.gov/Publications/osha3072.html*

25).   Answer A:

According to OSHA, "When testing for atmospheric hazards, a contractor should first test for oxygen. Combustible gas meters are oxygen-dependent and will not work properly in an oxygen-deficient atmosphere. Second, a contractor should test for combustible gases and vapors because the threat of fire or explosion is usually more immediate and life threatening. Third, a contractor must test for toxic gases and vapors."

https://www.osha.gov/dte/grant_materials/fy09/sh-18796-09/confinedspace.pdf

Domain 1: Quiz 6 Questions

1). What instrument would you use to measure an individual worker's TWA noise exposure?

    A) Noise Dosimeter.
    B) Sound meter.
    C) A dBA meter.
    D) A meter that measures in millibars.

2). What is the order of precedence for returning a locked-out machine to operation? Ensure the machine is:

    A) Clear of workers, fully assembled, controls in neutral, clear of tag/lock.
    B) Fully assembled, clear of workers, controls in neutral, clear of tag/lock.
    C) Controls in neutral, clear of workers, fully assembled, clear of tag/lock.
    D) Fully assembled, controls in neutral, clear of workers, clear of tag/lock.

3). Which activity increases the health hazards of asbestos?

    A) Scuba diving.
    B) Spelunking.
    C) Smoking.
    D) Sky diving.

4). How many wires may be broken in one lay of a wire rope sling before the sling is taken out of service?

    A) If five randomly distributed wires in one lay are broken.
    B) If ten randomly distributed wires in one lay are broken.
    C) If fifteen randomly distributed wires in one lay are broken.
    D) If twenty randomly distributed wires in one lay are broken.

5). In addition to prolonged exposure to Sunlight, what else might cause Dermatosis?

    A) Wearing long-sleeve shirts.
    B) Contact with chemicals.
    C) Washing the skin too often.
    D) Using too much barrier cream.

6).   What is the annual training requirement for confined space rescue team?
   A) CPR, entry training, rescue training.
   B) BCLS, CPR, entry training.
   C) Entry rescue training, CPR.
   D) BCLS, CPR, entry training, rescue training.

7).   The illustration shows the slope evacuation for what type of soil?
   A) Sand (type C soil).
   B) Silt (type B soil).
   C) Clay (type A soil).
   D) Rock.

8).   To reduce the risk of injury from Pneumatic tools, use:
   A) Air line for pressure relief if less than ½ in diameter.
   B) Positive locking device attaching the air hose to the tool.
   C) Air in the line at less than 32 psi.
   D) Electronic tools with GFCI – air tools are not allowed.

9).   Which air purifying cartridge would be the best to use for oil exposure?
   A) N100
   B) R100
   C) P100
   D) N95

10).   In addition to addressing cave-ins, which is the **greatest** concern with excavation or trenching operations?
   A) Heavy equipment operations across the job site 1000 feet away.
   B) A worker falls resulting in first aid treatment.
   C) Workers present in a hazardous atmosphere due to contaminated soil.
   D) Shoring and bracing is designed by a professional engineer.

11).   You have introduced ventilation that reduced a 100,000 PPM concentration of a flammable with LEL of 2.6% and UEL of 22% by 50%, is the concentration still flammable?
   A) Yes, because the concentration is 5%.
   B) Yes, because the concentration is 10%.
   C) No, the concentration is below the LEL.
   D) No, because it is still above the UEL.

12). When using a 2-leg, wire-rope sling with the angle between the sling legs and the load at 15 degrees, how much will the angle impact the allowed weight to be lifted?

    A) Increase it by 50%.
    B) No effect at all (90 degree angle).
    C) Reduce it by 50% (30 degree angle).
    D) Reduce it by 75%.

13). Which respirator offers the minimum APF for silica dust exposure during cutting operations?

    A) Air purifying half face.
    B) Air purifying full face.
    C) Air purifying full face negative pressure.
    D) Air purifying full face positive pressure.

14). What would be the best way to control the hazard exposure from a very loud piece of machinery?

    A) Move the machine further away from workers.
    B) Protect workers with hearing protection.
    C) Limit the time workers are in the area.
    D) Isolate the machine by placing it inside a structure.

15). Of the most common types of slings used in hoist operations, which is best to use with loads that are very hot?

    A) Synthetic.
    B) Wire rope.
    C) Chain.
    D) Mesh.

16). What does the illustrated crane hand signals indicate?

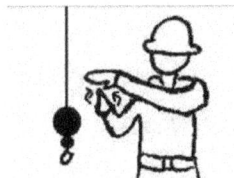

    A) All stop / emergency stop.
    B) Move slowly.
    C) Retract boom.
    D) Hoist (raise the load up).

17). Which lists the six most common types of asbestos found in the workplace?
    A) Chrysotile, Crocidolite, Actinolite, Amosite, Anthophyllite, Tremolite.
    B) Chrysotile, Actinolite, Amosite, Anthophyllite, Tremolite, Troglodyte.
    C) Chrysotile, Crocidolite, Actinolite, Ammonite, Anthophyllite, Tremolite.
    D) Chrysotile, Crocidolite, Actinolite, Anthophyllite, Tremolite, Trilobite.

18). What type of soil is **most** fine?
    A) Silt.
    B) Sand.
    C) Peat.
    D) Clay.

19). Of the **most** common types of slings used in hoist operations, which is **best** to use with delicate or easily damaged loads?
    A) Synthetic.
    B) Wire rope.
    C) Chain.
    D) Mesh.

20). Which is an example of a freezing injury?
    A) Hypothermia.
    B) Chilblains.
    C) Frostbite.
    D) Trench foot.

21). What is the **first** consideration for setting up for overhead crane operations?
    A) Establishing traffic control around the rig.
    B) Restricting parking around the rig.
    C) Electrical hazards overhead.
    D) Establishing the office trailer to direct the work.

22). What would be the **primary** concern when removing old paint?
 A) Lead.
 B) Asbestos.
 C) Solvent vapors.
 D) Simple dust exposure from particulates

23). What does the illustrated crane hand signals indicate?

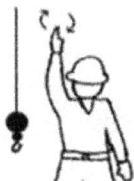

 A) Crew meeting (rally up)
 B) Move slowly
 C) Extend boom
 D) Hoist (raise the load up)

24). Which of these is **NOT** a common type of asbestos found in the workplace?
 A) Chrysotile (white asbestos - often contaminated with trace amounts of Tremolite).
 B) Amosite (brown asbestos).
 C) Crocidolite (blue asbestos).
 D) Aligalite (black asbestos).

25). When does the entry supervisor fill out the confined space entry permit?
 A) During the morning briefing.
 B) At the end of the previous day to be prepared for the next day.
 C) Just before any entry.
 D) After all conditions for entry have been met.

Domain 1: Quiz 6 Answers

1). Answer A:

According to OSHA's Technical Manual Section III: Chapter 5, a noise dosimeter can be used for "…averaging noise exposure over time and reporting results such as a TWA exposure or a percentage of the PEL".

2). Answer B:

Restoring Equipment to Service. When the servicing or maintenance is completed, and the machine or equipment is ready to return to normal operating condition, the following steps shall be taken.

(1) Check the machine or equipment and the immediate area around the machine to ensure that nonessential items have been removed and that the machine or equipment components are operationally intact.

(2) Check the work area to ensure that all employees have been safely positioned or removed from the area.

(3) Verify that the controls are in neutral.

(4) Remove the lockout devices and reenergize the machine or equipment.

https://www.osha.gov/pls/oshaweb/owadisp.show_document?p_table=STANDARDS&p_id=9805

3). Answer C:

Asbestos affects the body in the lungs. Asbestos fibers enter the lung and cause long-term issues with the lungs ability to infuse blood cells with oxygen. The main hazard associated with scuba diving would be an embolism from being submerged too long or ascending too quickly. The main hazard faced during spelunking (exploring caves) would be a "caught in" situation or crushed from a cavern collapse. The main hazard from sky diving would be an impact injury during landing—either with an open parachute or a catastrophic impact from a failed parachute. Smoking introduces contaminants directly to the lung tissue which would exacerbate the effects of an asbestos exposure.

4). Answer B:

The OSHA Pub 3072, Sling Safety, states for Wire Rope Sling Inspection "Wire rope slings must be visually inspected before each day's use. The operator should check the twists or lay of the sling. **If ten randomly**

---

distributed wires in one lay are broken, or five wires in one strand of a rope lay are damaged, the sling must not be used. It is not sufficient, however, to check only the condition of the wire rope. End fittings and other components should also be inspected for any damage that could make the sling unsafe."

https://www.osha.gov/Publications/osha3072.html

5).   Answer B:

According to many sources, dermatosis is a skin condition that doesn't involve inflammation. Skin conditions that involve inflammation is Dermatitis. Dermatosis usually results from exposure to many sources including sunlight and chemicals. Dermatitis differs from Dermatosis in that it is typically from one acute exposure. Example, Solar Dermatitis (Sunburn) results from an acute exposure to direct sunlight; however, photosensitive dermatosis (dermatosis from the sun) is considered a cutaneous disease that is generally the result of prolonged exposure to many factors which could include medications, other internal diseases/disorders, or immune considerations. Likewise, dermatosis from chemicals also results from prolonged exposure over time where the skin develops a sensitivity due to exposure over time.

6).   Answer A:

OSHA's Publication 3138 for Permit-Required Confined Spaces states "The standard requires employers to ensure that responders are capable of responding to an emergency in a timely manner. Employers must provide rescue service personnel with personal protective and rescue equipment, including respirators, and training in how to use it. Rescue service personnel also must receive the authorized entrants training and be trained to perform assigned rescue duties. The standard also requires that all rescuers be trained in first aid and CPR. At a minimum, one rescue team member must be currently certified in first aid and CPR. Employers must ensure that practice rescue exercises are performed yearly and that rescue services are provided access to permit spaces so they can practice rescue operations. Rescuers also must be informed of the hazards of the permit space."

7).   Answer A:

OSHA's Technical Manual covers the slope requirements for excavations as follows:

Soil Type	Height/Depth ratio	Slope Angle
Stable Rock	Vertical	90 deg.
Type A	¾ : 1	53 deg.
Type B	1 : 1	45 deg.
Type C	1½ : 1	34 deg.

https://www.osha.gov/dts/osta/otm/otm_v/otm_v_2.html

8). Answer B:

According to OSHA Pub 3080, "Hand and Powered Tools" "There are several dangers associated with the use of pneumatic tools. First and foremost is the danger of getting hit by one of the tool's attachments or by some kind of fastener the worker is using with the tool.

Pneumatic tools must be checked to see that the tools are fastened securely to the air hose to prevent them from becoming disconnected. A short wire or positive locking device attaching the air hose to the tool must also be used and will serve as an added safeguard.

If an air hose is more than 1 /2-inch (12.7 millimeters) in diameter, a safety excess flow valve must be installed at the source of the air supply to reduce pressure in case of hose failure. In general, the same precautions should be taken with an air hose that are recommended for electric cords, because the hose is subject to the same kind of damage or accidental striking, and because it also presents tripping hazards."

When using pneumatic tools, a safety clip or retainer must be installed to prevent attachments such as chisels on a chipping hammer from being ejected during tool operation.

9).   Answer C:

OSHA has accepted NIOSH's three categories of filter (N, R, and P), each with three levels of filter efficiency (95%, 99%, and 99.97%) for a total of nine respirator classes. The three levels of filter efficiency include the Type 100 (99.97% efficient), Type 99 (99% efficient), and the Type 95 (95% efficient). The classes of these air-purifying, particulate respirators certified under this classification are described in 42 CFR Part 84 Subpart K. (Volume 60 of the Federal Register page 30338, June 8, 1995.) This classification applies only to non-powered (negative pressure) respirators. Respirators certified under this classification replace the dust; dust, mist, fume; and HEPA respirators previously certified under 30 CFR Part 11. For powered air purifying respirators (PAPRs), HEPA filters remain available (42 CFR Part 84 Subpart kk).

Additional questions have been raised about which class of respirator should be used where a OSHA standard requires the use of a respirator with HEPA filters. Where workers are exposed to a hazard that would require the use of a respirator with HEPA filters the appropriate class of respirator under the 42 CFR Part 84 certification would be the Type 100. NIOSH has presently designated only the P100 respirator with the magenta color coding. However, the N100, R100, or P100 respirators have been certified at the 99.97% efficiency level and are identified as HEPA respirators.

Users are cautioned to note that the respirator classes are designated for use in certain environments with the P100 being the most universal (hence NIOSH's magenta color coding). Under these classes of respirators, if oil particles are present, users of respirators must refer to the following guide:
N series -- Not resistant to oil
R series -- Resistant to oil
P series -- oil Proof

10).   Answer C:

Hazardous Atmosphere is an atmosphere that by reason of being explosive, flammable, poisonous, corrosive, oxidizing, irritating, oxygen-deficient, toxic, or otherwise harmful may cause death, illness, or injury to persons exposed to it.

Workers exposed to the hazardous atmosphere during an excavation or trenching operations represents the greatest hazard.

11). Answer A:

100,000 PPM is equal to 10%. (Hint: A short cut when converting Parts Per Million-PPM to a percentage concentration is to remember 10,000 PPM equals a 1% concentration) A 50% reduction of 10% would still leave a concentration of 5%, which is still 2.4% above the LEL of 2.6%.

12). Answer D:

For sling lifts, remember the mnemonic "Double Divided Slings are Sinful". This is to remind you to divide twice to determine the stress on the sling leg. You divide once by the number of sling legs and then by the Sine of the angle of the sling legs. With an angle of 15 degrees, any load to be lifted will be divided by the Sine of 15, which is 0.2588, to determine the stress. This .2588 means the sling angle of 15 degrees will decrease the weight allowed to be lifted by about 75%.

13). Answer A:

According to 1926.1153 *"Respirable crystalline silica"*, the table *Specified Exposure Control Methods When Working with Materials Containing Crystalline Silica* specifies an APF of at least 10 when using PPE as a protection method.

According to OSHA's Respirable Crystalline Silica Standard for Construction, the Required Respiratory Protection and Minimum Assigned Protection Factor (APF) is 10, which equates to an Air-purifying, half mask respirator.

14). Answer D:

While isolation is not a specific category in the hierarchy of controls, the isolation option is the best course of action listed in the answer choices. Moving the machine is increasing distance—OSHA considers distance an administrative control. Hearing protection is PPE (the last option in the hierarchy). Limiting worker's time being exposed is considered an administrative control as well. Isolating the machine indicates some design and engineering action being taken with a newly built structure.

15). Answer C:

OSHA pub 3072 Sling Safety states "Chain slings are the best choice for lifting very hot materials. They can be heated to temperatures of up to 1,000°

Fahrenheit (538° centigrade); however, when alloy chain slings are consistently exposed to service temperatures more than 600° Fahrenheit (3 16° centigrade), operators must reduce the working load limits in accordance with the manufacturer's recommendations."   *https://www.osha.gov/Publications/osha3072.html*

16).   Answer B:

The hand signal of moving an upright hand slowly under an outstretched hand is the signal for the crane operator to move the load slowly. Learn all the hand and arm signals as covered by Appendix A to Subpart CC of Part 1926--Standard Hand Signals.

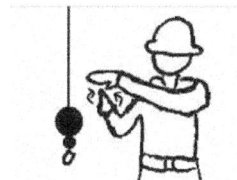

17).   Answer A:

The six most common types of asbestos found in the workplace are Chrysotile, Crocidolite, Actinolite, Amosite, Anthophyllite, Tremolite. A Troglogyte is a term used to describe a hermit, recluse or person who is regarded as being deliberately ignorant or old-fashioned, a "cave dweller". An Ammonite is a widely known fossil, with a ribbed spiral-form shell. Trilobites are a fossil group of extinct marine arthropods.

18).   Answer D:

The coarseness of soil is important in trenching or digging because that impacts the soil's stability and the potential for collapse. Soil coarseness runs from Sand, which is very coarse to Clay which is not.

19).   Answer A:

OSHA pub 3072 Sling Safety states "Fiber rope and synthetic web slings are used primarily for temporary work, such as construction and painting jobs, and in marine operations. They also are the best choice for use on expensive loads, highly finished parts, fragile parts, and delicate equipment."

20).   Answer C:

Frostbite is a **freezing** injury. Hypothermia is a condition of an abnormally low core body temperature—usually below 95.0 °F. Chilblains is a condition from repeated or prolonged exposure to cold air (not freezing air) that results in the skin's small blood vessels becoming inflamed. Trench foot is a condition of the feet from prolonged exposure to damp and cold conditions.

21). Answer C:

According to OSHA, more than half of overhead crane accidents are the result of encountering some sort of electrical hazards. These events often result in serious, and often fatal injuries.

22). Answer A:

OSHA States "Plumbers, welders, and painters are among those workers most exposed to lead. Significant lead exposures also can arise from removing paint from surfaces previously coated with lead-based paint such as bridges, residences being renovated, and structures being demolished or salvaged. With the increase in highway work, bridge repair, residential lead abatement, and residential remodeling, the potential for exposure to lead-based paint has become more common."
-https://www.osha.gov/Publications/osha3142.pdf

23). Answer D:

The hand signal of a raised hand above the head, moving in a circular motion indicates the crane operator to raise the load up. Learn all the hand and arm signals as covered by Appendix A to Subpart CC of Part 1926--Standard Hand Signals.

24). Answer D:

Chrysotile, Amosite and Crocidolite are all types of asbestos found in industry. Aligalite is a totally fictional term playing on the real "Crocidolite" similarities with Crocodile and combining Alligator with an asbestos sounding ending.

25). Answer D:

Of all the options offered, the best answer is "after all conditions for entry have been met". For more information, see OSHA Publication 3138 Permit-Required Confined Spaces.

Domain 1: Quiz 7 Questions

1). What is the **primary** hazard to crane operators during crane operations?
   A) High winds.
   B) Uneven terrain.
   C) Electrical hazards.
   D) MSDs from operating the controls.

2). Of the **most common** types of slings used in hoist operations, which is best to use with loads that have sharp edges?
   A) Synthetic.
   B) Wire rope.
   C) Chain.
   D) Mesh.

3). Which of these accounts for up to 95% of asbestos used in U.S. buildings today?
   A) Chrysotile Asbestos.
   B) Tremolite Asbestos.
   C) Amosite Asbestos.
   D) Crocidolite Asbestos.

4). What would be the **primary** exposure concern when using a cutting torch on an old painted metal structure?
   A) Asbestos.
   B) Slag.
   C) Lead.
   D) Skin exposure to heat.

5). What hazardous substance may a worker encounter during a remodel of an old building is of **greatest** concern?
   A) Asbestos.
   B) Dry Wall.
   C) Solar panels.
   D) Treated lumber.

6). What is the minimum requirements for Confined space entry?
   A) Atmospheric testing, permit, rescue.
   B) Permit, attendant, insurance.
   C) Rescue, atmospheric testing, attendant.
   D) Supervisor, attendant, permit.

7). When using an Oxy-acetylene torch, the hose shall be:
   A) Selected based on the pressure setting you are going to use.
   B) A combined hose so the gasses are mixed in the hose.
   C) Left in service even if they have damage if they don't leak.
   D) Easily distinguishable between the fuel gas hose and oxygen hose.

8). What is the hood air flow rate for ventilation during silica sand blasting?
   A) 20 CFM.
   B) 50 CFM.
   C) 80 CFM.
   D) 100 CFM.

9). What is the APF rating of an air purifying half-face respirator compared to a throw-away mask?
   A) The dust mask's APF is 1/10th the half-face respirator.
   B) The half-face is 10 times better than the dust mask.
   C) They both have an APF of 10.
   D) The dust mask's APF is 10 but the half-face's APF is 100.

10). What would be the **primary** concern for employees entering an area with a high concentration of rodent droppings?
   A) Legionnaire's disease.
   B) Hantavirus.
   C) Bubonic plague.
   D) Smallpox.

11). What would be your greatest concern (priority) if you learned of all these following happening at the same time—which should you handle **first**?
   A) Supervisor in a vehicle accident but is uninjured.
   B) Trench with partial cave in with no injuries.
   C) Five workers on the 5th floor with no fall protection.
   D) Workers cutting concrete being exposed to silica dust.

12). Which of these is an example of passive fall protection system?
   A) PFAS.
   B) Restraint system.
   C) Warning lines / temporary railing.
   D) Posted signs.

13). What is the maximum wind speed for work on a suspended scaffold?
   A) 20 mph.
   B) 25 mph.
   C) 30 mph.
   D) 35 mph.

14). What fall protection device would you use to absorb the energy of arresting an employee's fall?
   A) Retractable lanyard.
   B) Shock lanyard.
   C) Engineered anchor points.
   D) Body belts.

15). What is the first thing to consider when you have employees who are going to use a PFAS?
   A) Suspended worker rescue.
   B) Body belt fitting.
   C) Warning signs.
   D) Harness / lanyard compatibility.

16). What are generally the two kinds of barricades used in construction?
   A) Active / passive.
   B) General / specific.
   C) Hard / soft.
   D) Warning / caution.

17). The CHST notices contractors about to energize a newly installed piece of equipment for first time on a crowded multi-employer work site, which is **best** course of action?
   A) Delay start up.
   B) Ignore it.
   C) Ask non-involved workers to leave.
   D) Note it for a discussion topic at the next shift briefing.

18). Which is an example of a "caught in between" hazard?
   A) Being hit by a crane hook.
   B) Being struck by a falling tool from a scaffold.
   C) Striking your thumb with a hammer.
   D) Being pinned by a rotating crane body.

19). You notice the body of a crane is in tight spot up with only 1' clearance from building, what would you do?
    A) Have the operator relocate the crane to an area that isn't good for the lift but will provide more clearance to the building.
    B) Suspend crane operations.
    C) Recommend to the crane operator to protect the rear swing radius with barriers to prevent someone from being caught in between the crane body and the building.
    D) Document the situation in your daily report.

20). Before energizing equipment on a cut lock procedure, what is the most important to do?
    A) Notify affected workers.
    B) Clear the machine of tools, equipment and people.
    C) Verify energy is controlled.
    D) Preserve the original lock as evidence.

21). What are the concerns with a class 2 laser?
    A) Not known to cause eye injury.
    B) Cannot emit laser radiation at known hazard levels.
    C) Hazardous for intra-beam viewing.
    D) Hazardous to view under any condition.

22). Surveyor is setting up a laser on crowded job site, what to do?
    A) Suspend work and clear area.
    B) Ask the surveyor to delay his work until your crew is finished for the day.
    C) Report the surveyor to OSHA for exposing your crew to laser hazards.
    D) Go speak with the surveyor to see if controls are needed to prevent potential exposures based on the equipment he is using.

23). An example of a chronic exposure is:
    A) Mesothelioma.
    B) Fainting/dizziness from a drop in blood pressure.
    C) Heat Stroke.
    D) Metal Fume Fever.

24). How long does an employer have to keep confined space entry permits?
    A) Only until the end of the workday the entry is made.
    B) Only until the completion of that job/project.
    C) 1 year.
    D) 30 years.

25). For electrical safety on construction sites, OSHA requires employers to ensure either a scheduled and recorded assured equipment grounding conductor program or:
    A) UL certified extension cords.
    B) That all electrical tools have grounding (3-prong) plugs.
    C) That all electrical tools are double insulated.
    D) GFCIs for receptacle outlets in use.

26). What is required to be on an entry permit for confined space?
    A) Name of job site where permit space to be entered.
    B) Equipment used to test for hazards.
    C) Date and authorized duration of the last time someone made entry.
    D) Any other information needed to ensure employee safety.

27). What type of soil is sand?
    A) Type A.
    B) Type B.
    C) Type C.
    D) Stable Rock.

28). What does the illustrated crane hand signals indicate?

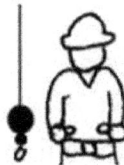

    A) All stop / emergency stop.
    B) Outriggers in.
    C) Retract boom.
    D) Chocks in.

Domain 1: Quiz 7 Answers

1). Answer C:

According to OSHA, more than half of overhead crane accidents are the result of coming into contact with some sort of electrical hazards. These events often result in serious, and often fatal injuries.

2). Answer D:

We chose 'Mesh' because for loads that have sharp edges, a wire mesh sling is best to use because of its durability and multiple touch points with the sharp edges of the load.

3). Answer A:

While the answer options are all real types of asbestos, Chrysotile accounts for the vast majority of all asbestos in U.S. buildings today.

4). Answer C:

OSHA States "Plumbers, welders, and painters are among those workers most exposed to lead. Significant lead exposures also can arise from removing paint from surfaces previously coated with lead-based paint such as bridges, residences being renovated, and structures being demolished or salvaged. With the increase in highway work, bridge repair, residential lead abatement, and residential remodeling, the potential for exposure to lead-based paint has become more common." *-https://www.osha.gov/Publications/osha3142.pdf*

5). Answer A:

The OSHA Fact Sheet on Asbestos states that the asbestos "…hazard may occur during manufacturing of asbestos-containing products; performing brake or clutch repairs; renovating or demolishing buildings or ships; or cleanup from those activities; contact with deteriorating asbestos containing materials and during cleanup after natural disasters."

6). Answer A:

There are many requirements to ensure personnel are safe when entering a confined space, however, of the options offered here the BEST answer is at a minimum, employers will have a permit process, have ensured the atmosphere is safe and ensure there is a rescue process established prior to allowing anyone to enter the space. *https://www.osha.gov/dte/grant_materials/fy09/sh-18796-09/confinedspace.pdf*

7).   Answer D:

The specification for oxyacetylene torch hoses is found in the Compressed Gas Association (CGA) and RMA (Rubber Manufacturer's Association) <u>Specification for Rubber Welding Hose</u> (1958). The requirements of this standard is incorporated into 1910.253 by reference (1910.6). It specifies that the hoses will be easily distinguishable between each other, they must be separate so the gases are not mixed until the nozzle and they are rated for a specific pressure regardless the regulator setting. **In addition, 1910.253(e)(5)(v) states "Hose showing leaks, burns, worn places, or other defects rendering it unfit for service shall be repaired or replaced."**

8).   Answer C:

According to the CDC's <u>Industrial Health and Safety Criteria for Abrasive Blast Cleaning Operations</u>, "For adequate dust clearance, a minimum air flow rate of approximately 20 CFM/FT2 should be used with non-silica abrasives. Higher mnl1mum rates should be used with low density or toxic abrasives that exhibit a tendency 2 to fracture extensively. For example, past experience has shown 80 CFM/FT to be effective for the control of silica sand dust.
Cross draft ventilation is effective both in totally enclosed abrasive blasting facilities and in semi-enclosed abrasive blasting facilities. Air flow rates should be in the same range (preferably higher) but no lower than t hose for downdraft systems designed for identical operating conditions. Up flow ventilation should not be used in abrasive blasting enclosures."

9).   Answer C:

According to OSHA's Publication 3352 "Assigned Protection Factors for the Revised Respiratory Protection Standard", both a half-mask Air-purifying respirator (APR) AND a "Half mask/Dust mask" have an Assigned Protection Factor (APF) of 10.

10).   Answer B:

According to the Center for Disease Control (CDC), people could get Hantavirus Pulmonary Syndrome (HPS) when they breathe in Hantaviruses. Hantaviruses could be present in rodent urine and droppings and can be spread when those droppings or dried urine residue that contains a Hantavirus are stirred up into the air. The CDC's summary <u>Facts About Hantaviruses</u> states: "People can also become infected when they touch mouse or rat urine, droppings, or nesting materials that contain the virus and then touch their eyes, nose, or mouth. They can also get HPS from a mouse or rat bite."

11). Answer C:

Often safety personnel are faced with competing priorities and must choose which actions take precedence. Workers five floors above ground level with no fall protection are exposed to an immediately dangerous and life threatening situation. The next item of concern might be the partial cave-in IF there are still personnel in the trench. If not, the silica exposure is an important concern due to the long-term impact of silica on the lungs. The vehicle accident is the least concerning as it has already happened so the safety person can do nothing to mitigate it at all.

12). Answer C:

Fall protection is generally discussed by OSHA as restraint or arrest (PFAS=Personal Fall Arrest System). An arrest system is a PPE based system which stops an employee in the air and suspends them above the ground after they have fallen over an unprotected edge. A restraint system is a PPE based system which restricts the employee so they cannot fall over an unprotected edge. The best protection is a guard rail or other means limiting an employee's approach to the actual fall hazard. The industry will refer to these as passive fall protection systems. A posted sign is just a warning and is not considered fall protection at all.

13). Answer B:

1926.451(f)(12) states "Work on or from scaffolds is prohibited during storms or high winds unless a competent person has determined that it is safe for employees to be on the scaffold and those employees are protected by a personal fall arrest system or wind screens. Wind screens shall not be used unless the scaffold is secured against the anticipated wind forces imposed."

1910.66(i)(2)(v) states "The platform shall not be operated in winds in excess of 25 miles per hour (40.2 km/hr) except to move it from an operating to a storage position. Wind speed shall be determined based on the best available information, which includes on-site anemometer readings and local weather forecasts which predict wind velocities for the area."

14). Answer B:

Of the options listed, the only one which would absorb any of the energy generated during a fall would be a shock lanyard. A shock lanyard is a lanyard which is specifically designed to lessen the impact of the stress of the arrest by either incorporating elastic material or sewn folds of material which rip apart in a controlled fashion during the arrest to slow the arrest and spread the 'stopping' action over time so the individual does not experience the impact all at once.

15). Answer A:

1926.502(d)(20) states "The employer shall provide for prompt rescue of employees in the event of a fall or shall assure that employees are able to rescue themselves." Because this is often overlooked and an arrested worker left suspended for an extended period of time could result in permanent damage, rescue is considered the first concern to work out when employing a personal fall arrest system (PFAS).

16). Answer C:

Soft barricades use some sort of wire rope or tape as safety barriers to prevent or restrict access to an area. They are usually used where physical protection is not needed.

Hard barricades are usually self-supporting such as concrete, plastic, or other solid barriers. They are usually placed to physically restrict entry of persons to an area.

17). Answer C:

Any potential hazard exposure should never be ignored. Some pre-emptive action should always be taken to avoid the exposure and to increase awareness among the employee population. Interrupting the operation (Delaying the start-up) is always an option, but often there are other options that may accomplish the same outcome. Presumably, the workers which need to be there have been trained on the equipment's characteristics and potential hazards so by asking all workers who are not involved to leave the area would accomplish the same outcome as a delay without delaying the schedule.

18). Answer D:

Caught in between hazards are when the worker is pressed from both sides or from one side into or against another surface as sort. These are characterized by action verbs like "caught, pinned, crushed, squeezed", etcetera. The other options of "hit by a crane", "struck by a falling tool", or "hitting a body part with a hammer" are all examples of "Struck by" injuries.

19). Answer C:

The best option of the ones offered would be to establish a warning zone around the hazard area. Although this is an administrative control, it is better than suspending the operation or increasing hazards of a safe lift by relocating the crane.

20). Answer B:

1910.147(e)(3) states "Lockout or tagout devices removal. Each lockout or tagout device shall be removed from each energy isolating device by the employee who applied the device. Exception to paragraph (e)(3): When the authorized employee who applied the lockout or tagout device is not available to remove it, that device may be removed under the direction of the employer, provided that specific procedures and training for such removal have been developed, documented and incorporated into the employer's energy control program. The employer shall demonstrate that the specific procedure provides equivalent safety to the removal of the device by the authorized employee who applied it. The specific procedure shall include at least the following elements: (3)(i) Verification by the employer that the authorized employee who applied the device is not at the facility: 3)(ii) Making all reasonable efforts to contact the authorized employee to inform him/her that his/her lockout or tagout device has been removed; and (3)(iii) Ensuring that the authorized employee has this knowledge before he/she resumes work at that facility.

21). Answer A:

OSHA Technical Manual, Section 3, Chapter 6 covers laser classifications:

Class I: cannot emit laser radiation at known hazard levels (typically continuous wave: cw 0.4 µW at visible wavelengths). Users of Class I laser products are generally exempt from radiation hazard controls during operation and maintenance (but not necessarily during service).

Since lasers are not classified on beam access during service, most Class I industrial lasers will consist of a higher class (high power) laser enclosed in a properly interlocked and labeled protective enclosure. In some cases, the enclosure may be a room (walk-in protective housing) which requires a means to prevent operation when operators are inside the room.

Class I.A.: a special designation that is based upon a 1000-second exposure and applies only to lasers that are "not intended for viewing" such as a supermarket laser scanner. The upper power limit of Class I.A. is 4.0 mW. The emission from a Class I.A. laser is defined such that the emission does not exceed the Class I limit for an emission duration of 1000 seconds.

Class II: low-power visible lasers that emit above Class I levels but at a radiant power not above 1 mW. The concept is that the human aversion reaction to bright light will protect a person. Only limited controls are specified.

Class IIIA: intermediate power lasers (cw: 1-5 mW). Only hazardous for intrabeam viewing. Some limited controls are usually recommended.

> *NOTE*: There are different logotype labeling requirements for Class IIIA lasers with a beam irradiance that does not exceed 2.5 mW/cm^2 (Caution logotype) and those where the beam irradiance does exceed 2.5 mW/cm^2 (Danger logotype).

Class IIIB: moderate power lasers (cw: 5-500 mW, pulsed: 10 J/cm^2 or the diffuse reflection limit, whichever is lower). In general Class IIIB lasers will not be a fire hazard, nor are they generally capable of producing a hazardous diffuse reflection. Specific controls are recommended.

Class IV: High power lasers (cw: 500 mW, pulsed: 10 J/cm^2 or the diffuse reflection limit) are hazardous to view under any condition (directly or diffusely scattered) and are a potential fire hazard and a skin hazard. Significant controls are required of Class IV laser facilities

22).   Answer D:

Of the options given, speaking with the surveyor about the potential exposures is the BEST course of action. Assuming you know the hazards is a frequent—and arrogant—action many safety people take. You will often find a simple conversation will pay benefits well beyond the immediate concern the situation may involve.

23). Answer A:

According to the Department of Health and Human Services, "Chemical exposures are generally divided into two categories: acute and chronic. The term "chronic exposure" generally refers to exposures to "low" concentrations of a contaminant over a long period of time. The "low" concentrations required to produce symptoms of chronic exposure depend upon the chemical, the duration of each exposure, and the number of exposures." (Occupational Safety and Health Guidance Manual for Hazardous Waste Site Activities) Fainting, heat stroke and metal fume fever are all the result of a short-term exposure or event. Mesothelioma is a cancer of mesothelial tissue, typically associated with exposure to asbestos inhaled into the lungs over time.

24). Answer C:

1910.146(e)(6) states: "The employer shall retain each canceled entry permit for at least 1 year to facilitate the review of the permit-required confined space program required by paragraph (d)(14) of this section. Any problems encountered during an entry operation shall be noted on the pertinent permit so that appropriate revisions to the permit space program can be made.
"NOTE: Employers may perform a single annual review covering all entries performed during a 12-month period. If no entry is performed during a 12-month period, no review is necessary."

You may discard the cancelled entry permits after the review. However, keep in mind that OSHA's standard on access to employee exposure and medical records (1910.1020) requires the employer to maintain employee exposure records for at least 30 years. If you needed to monitor the entrants' exposure to toxic substances during the entry, OSHA expects you to keep a record of this exposure - see 1910.1020(d)(1)(ii) and 1910.1020(c)(5).

25). Answer D:

OSHA ground-fault protection rules and regulations have been determined necessary and appropriate for employee safety and health. Therefore, it is the employer's responsibility to provide either: (a) GFCIs on construction sites for receptacle outlets in use and not part of the permanent wiring of the building or structure; or (b) a scheduled and recorded assured equipment grounding conductor program on construction sites, covering all cord sets, receptacles which are not part of the permanent wiring of the building or structure, and equipment connected by cord and plug which are available for use or used by employees.

The employer is required to provide approved GFCIs for all 120-volt, single-phase, 15- and 20-ampere receptacle outlets on construction sites that are not a part of the permanent wiring of the building or structure and that are in use by employees. If a receptacle or receptacles are installed as part of the permanent wiring of the building or structure and they are used for temporary electric power, GFCI protection shall be provided. Receptacles on the ends of extension cords are not part of the permanent wiring and, therefore the cord's receptacle, must be of the GFCI type whether or not the extension cord is plugged into permanent wiring. These GFCIs monitor the current-to-the-load for leakage to ground.

https://www.osha.gov/Publications/3007/3007.html

26).   Answer D:

According to OHSA, Entry permits must include:
- Name of permit space to be entered, authorized entrant(s), eligible attendants and individuals authorized to be entry supervisors;
- Test results;
- Tester's initials or signature;
- Name and signature of supervisor who authorizes entry;
- Purpose of entry and known space hazards;
- Measures to be taken to isolate permit spaces and to eliminate or control space hazards;
- Name and telephone numbers of rescue and emergency services and means to be used to contact them;
- Date and authorized duration of entry;
- Acceptable entry conditions;
- Communication procedures and equipment to maintain contact during entry;
- Additional permits, such as for hot work, that have been issued authorizing work in the permit space;
- Special equipment and procedures, including personal protective equipment and alarm systems; and
- Any other information needed to ensure employee safety.

27). Answer C:

We chose answer C because: OSHA categorizes soil and rock deposits into four types, Stable Rock and Type A through C.

Stable Rock is natural solid mineral matter that can be excavated with vertical sides and remain intact while exposed. It is usually identified by a rock name such as granite or sandstone. Determining whether a deposit is of this type may be difficult unless it is known whether cracks exist and whether or not the cracks run into or away from the excavation.

Type A Soils are cohesive soils with an unconfined compressive strength of 1.5 tons per square foot (tsf) (144 kPa) or greater. Examples of Type A cohesive soils are often: clay, silty clay, sandy clay, clay loam and, in some cases, silty clay loam and sandy clay loam. (No soil is Type A if it is fissured, is subject to vibration of any type, has previously been disturbed, is part of a sloped, layered system where the layers dip into the excavation on a slope of 4 horizontal to 1 vertical (4H:1V) or greater, or has seeping water.

Type B Soils are cohesive soils with an unconfined compressive strength greater than 0.5 tsf (48 kPa) but less than 1.5 tsf (144 kPa). Examples of other Type B soils are: angular gravel; silt; silt loam; previously disturbed soils unless otherwise classified as Type C; soils that meet the unconfined compressive strength or cementation requirements of Type A soils but are fissured or subject to vibration; dry unstable rock; and layered systems sloping into the trench at a slope less than 4H:1V (only if the material would be classified as a Type B soil).

Type C Soils are cohesive soils with an unconfined compressive strength of 0.5 tsf (48 kPa) or less. Other Type C soils include granular soils such as gravel, sand and loamy sand, submerged soil, soil from which water is freely seeping, and submerged rock that is not stable. Also included in this classification is material in a sloped, layered system where the layers dip into the excavation or have a slope of four horizontal to one vertical (4H:1V) or greater.

Layered Geological Strata. Where soils are configured in layers, i.e., where a layered geologic structure exists, the soil must be classified on the basis of the soil classification of the weakest soil layer. Each layer may be classified individually if a more stable layer lies below a less stable layer, i.e., where a Type C soil rests on top of stable rock.

28).   Answer C:

Holding hands to the front at waist level, thumbs pointing towards each other with the fingers closed is the signal for retracting the boom.

Domain 2: Emergency Preparedness and Fire Prevention

Domain 2 *Emergency Preparedness and Fire Prevention • 10.3%*
Knowledge of:
1. Proper fire protection and prevention methods (e.g., appropriate class of fire extinguishers, inspection criteria)
2. Components of emergency action plans
3. Common elements of response plans for environmental hazards (e.g., releases or spills)
4. Emergency response system (e.g., incident command system, crisis management, emergency response equipment, media)
5. Potential first aid or medical needs (e.g., availability of first aid kit, AED, CPR supplies)
6. Universal precautions (e.g., bloodborne/airborne pathogens)
Skill to:
1. Plan for emergencies

Domain 2: Quiz 1 Questions

1). Which of the following firefighting agents has proven to be the most effective in combating Class B fires?
   A) Foam, CO_2, Dry Powder.
   B) AFFF, Halon, Dry Chemical.
   C) Halon, Water, Dry Chemical.
   D) Foam, CO_2, Dry Chemical.

2). The possibility of fire during construction operations is higher than during regular occupancy. Accordingly, storage of flammable liquid materials is strictly controlled on a construction site. Which of the following best describes the correct safety practices concerning storage of flammable/combustible liquids in a building under construction.
   A) Flammables stored inside not in an approved flammable storage cabinet are limited to 10 gallons.
   B) Flammables stored inside not in an approved flammable storage cabinet are limited to 25 gallons.
   C) Stairwell storage is limited to 60 gallons of flammables and 120 gallons of combustibles.
   D) Flammables cannot be stored on a construction site at any time, combustibles are limited to 10 gallons or a one-day supply whichever is less.

3). Which of the following correctly indicates the minimum access width leading to an exit required by the NFPA "Life Safety Code"?
   A) 32 inches.
   B) 22 inches.
   C) 28 inches.
   D) 36 inches.

4). What horizontal spacing is required between two ladders in a trench?
   A)   50 feet.
   B)   100 feet.
   C)   10 feet.
   D)   30 feet.

5). Self-contained breathing apparatus (SCBA) used as emergency or rescue equipment must be inspected on what frequency?
   A) Annually
   B) Semiannually
   C) Monthly
   D) Weekly

6). What characterizes a Class II, Division 2 location (according to the National Electrical Code)?
   A) A location where flammable or combustible vapors may be present in sufficient quantities to be hazardous
   B) A location where combustible dust is normally present in sufficient quantities to be hazardous
   C) A location where flammable or combustible vapors are not normally present, but might be due to abnormal or periodic operations
   D) A location where combustible dust is not normally present but might be due to abnormal or periodic operations

7). Lift trucks and manufacturing and information technology equipment are potential ignition sources that could cause a dust explosion or deflagration. What should SH&E professionals consider when evaluating ignition sources?
   A) Electrical machines
   B) Dust producing processes
   C) Class IV forklifts
   D) Several ignition sources

8). Entry into a confined space is required at one of your construction sites. The oxygen concentration in the confined space has been measured at 16%. Which of the following most correctly indicates the danger to personnel entering this atmosphere?
   A) 16% oxygen causes tingling in the fingers and toes
   B) This level of oxygen is adequate for rescue operations only
   C) Time spent in this atmosphere should be limited
   D) This level of oxygen could cause impairment of judgment and difficult breathing

9). A liquid with a flash point of 50°F and a boiling point of 110°F would be classified by the OSHA and the NFPA as a:
   A) Class I flammable liquid
   B) Class IA combustible liquid
   C) Class IB flammable liquid
   D) Class II combustible liquid

10). Investigation of a dust explosion involves determining the actual hazard as well as the manufacturing process that led to high dust concentration levels. What should SH&E professionals look for when evaluating a workplace?
   A) A documented process hazard analysis and operator training
   B) The physical and chemical properties that establish the hazardous characteristics of the materials used in a facility.
   C) Housekeeping and predictive/preventative maintenance programs
   D) All of these are important to an evaluation

11). Which of the following provides the best reason for not transporting flammable liquids in an approved safety can in the closed trunk of an automobile?
   A) Just not a good idea
   B) Can could tip over and spill
   C) Excessive heat could cause can to rupture
   D) Potential for vapor release from the can

12). When conducting a fire investigation, the number one area to be determined is?
   A) Fire ignition sequence
   B) Response time
   C) Number of deaths
   D) Were all building and fire codes followed in construction

13). The chance of a dust cloud igniting is governed by what?
   A) Oxygen content and dust accumulation
   B) Size of dust particles and impurities present
   C) Strength of the source of ignition
   D) All the above

14). What factors influence the destructiveness of dust explosions?
 A) Size of dust
 B) Amount of dust
 C) Pressure rise, pressure developed, duration etc.
 D) Confinement and mixture

15). A _____ is an object that connects a piece of electrical equipment to earth or some conducting body that serves in place of earth. A _____ serves to complete the electrical circuit and prevent the hazard to electrical shock caused by defective equipment and that may cause death or serious injury.
 A) Bond
 B) Ground
 C) Metal frame
 D) Double-insulation

16). On a construction site, at least one portable fire extinguisher having a rating of not less than 20-B units shall be located not less than ___ feet, nor more than ____ feet, from any flammable liquid storage area located outside.
 A) 25, 75
 B) 25, 100
 C) 50, 75
 D) 50, 100

17). How does the Hazard Communication Standard labeling requirement apply to industrial fire extinguishers?
 A) All fire extinguishers must be labeled
 B) Fire extinguishers containing compressed gas are required to be labeled
 C) Does not apply
 D) Only extinguishers containing hazardous agents over 20 lbs need to be labeled

18). Untrained personnel who are unfamiliar with the product or the hazards involved but who want to help in an emergency is a reason why the latches on the outside of aircraft to release cockpit canopies are marked. Which of the following is not true about such devices?
   A) Such devices must be foolproof in an emergency
   B) They require little physical effort to operate
   C) They can be easy to operate when only a few words of instruction are provided
   D) They must be labeled in multiple languages

19). Under ICS, the Command Staff positions include:
   A) Safety Officer, Public Information Officer, and Liaison Officer.
   B) Liaison Officer, Operations Section Chief, and Finance and Administration Section Chief.
   C) Public Information Officer, Chief Executive Officer, and Safety Officer.
   D) Logistics Section Chief, Safety Officer, and the Contracting Officer.

20). Multiple 60 gal flammable cabinets stored on a job site must be separated from a building under construction by?
   A) 20 feet
   B) 50' feet
   C) 75 feet
   D) 100 feet

21). In decontamination, the Contamination Reduction Zone is the area between the Hot Line and the:
   A) Exclusion Zone
   B) Contamination Control Line
   C) Access Control Point
   D) Contamination Reduction Corridor Line

22). What shape indicates the class of fire extinguisher is used for electrical fires?
   A) Triangle
   B) Square
   C) Circle
   D) Star

23). What does GHS stand for?
   A) Global Horizontal System
   B) Globally Hazard System
   C) Globally Harmonized System
   D) Global Honor System

24). Considering the five C's for ICS (command; control; communication; coordination; cooperation), which is the most important?
   A) Communication
   B) Coordination
   C) Cooperation
   D) Command

25). List the part of communication in order
   A) Sender – message – receiver – feedback
   B) Sender – receiver – message – feedback
   C) Receiver – message – sender – feedback
   D) Message – sender – receiver – feedback

Domain 2: Quiz 1 Answers

1). Answer D:

The most effective agents for Class B fires involving flammable liquids are Foam, CO_2, and Dry Chemical.

2). Answer B:

According to OSHA at 1926.152 no more than 25 gallons of flammable or combustible liquids can be stored inside without being in an approved storage cabinet or in a room specifically designed for the storage of flammables/combustibles. The quantity is incorrect in selection "A". Selection "C" incorrectly provides storage in stairwells, which is expressly prohibited. Selection "D" is both unrealistic and incorrect. **1910.1200(f)(5)** Except as provided in paragraphs (f)(6) and (f)(7) of this section, the employer shall ensure that each container of hazardous chemicals in the workplace is labeled, tagged or marked with the following information:

Identity of the hazardous chemical(s) contained therein; and appropriate hazard warnings, or alternatively, words, pictures, symbols, or combination thereof, which provide at least general information regarding the hazards of the chemicals, and which, in conjunction with the other information immediately available to employees under the hazard communication program, will provide employees with the specific information regarding the physical and health hazards of the hazardous chemical.

3). Answer C:

The minimum access to an exit required by NFPA 101 the "Life Safety Code" is 28 inches for "grandfathered" structures. New construction requires as minimum of 36 inches.

4). Answer A:

Means of egress from trench excavations such as a stairway, ladder, ramp or other safe means of egress are required in trench excavations that are 4 feet or more in depth and located so as to require **no more than 25 feet of lateral travel** for workers. Ladders placed every 50 running feet of trench would provide a maximum of 25 feet of travel in each direction, assuming an initial ladder at the start of the trench run. OSHA 1926.651.

5). Answer C:

OSHA requires monthly inspections for self-contained breathing apparatus.

6). Answer D:

Class II, Division 2 locations are those in which combustible dust is not normally present but might be due to abnormal or periodic operations. During those times, sufficient dust may be present in the air to produce explosive or ignitable mixtures. A Class II, Division 2 location is an area normally free of dust, but due to some incident, dust may be introduced. Mechanical breakdown of a valve or a break in a pipe are examples of conditions that would require an area to be classified as Division 2.

7). Answer D:

Several ignition sources can cause a dust explosion or deflagration. Primary sources of ignition include electrical; sparking from tramp metals or broken equipment pieces; heat from bearings, belts and misaligned buckets; improperly prepared maintenance and hot work operations; forklifts and vehicles; and natural causes, such as lightning. One of the first considerations is to identify the electrical classification of the area or room volume. NFPA70, the National Electrical Code (NEC), Chapter 5, Special Occupancies, addresses hazardous locations. It defines the classification of several special occupancies, such as flammable liquids, gases and vapors; combustible dusts; and other materials. It is meant to integrate with other NFPA standards that more fully address the particular occupancy. For electrical issues, the NEC defines what electrical devices are permitted in a given area. The definitions located in section 500.2 are important to know when addressing special occupancies. This section defines terms such as dust ignition-proof, dusttight, and purged and pressurized.

8).   Answer D:

OSHA requires 19.5% oxygen for all surface work. The scale below describes some problems associated with oxygen-deficient atmospheres.

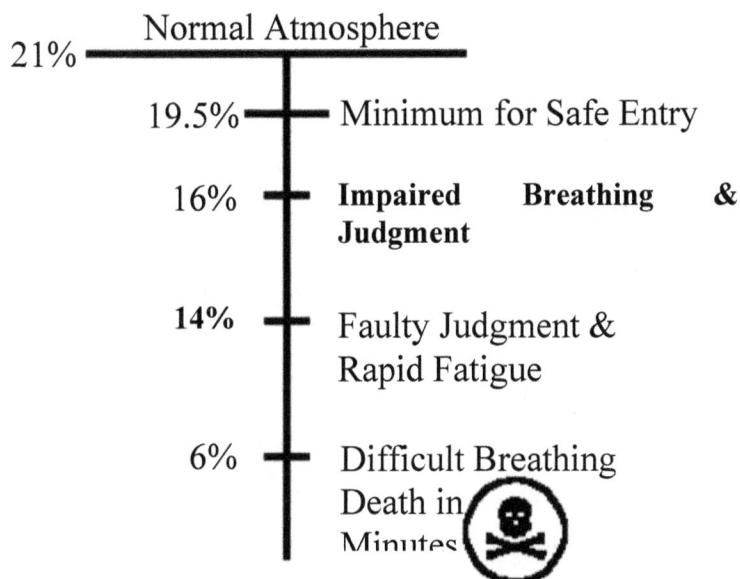

9).   Answer C:

Flammable and combustible liquids are subdivided into classes as shown below (taken from NFPA 30 and 321, *Basic Classification of Flammable and Combustible Liquids*).

FLAMMABLE			
CLASS		Boiling Point	Flash Point
I			below 100 F
IA		below 100 F	below 73 F
IB		at or above 100 F	below 73 F
IC			at or above 73 F and below 100 F
COMBUSTIBLE			
II			at or above 100 F and below 140 F
III			at or above 140 F
III A			at or above 140 F and below 200 F
III B			at or above 200 F

Note: When a combustible liquid is heated to within 30°F of its flashpoint, it must be classified and handled in accordance with the next lowest class of liquid.

10). Answer D:

SH&E professionals should be thoroughly familiar with the processes and facilities that handle combustible particulate solids in a facility. They also should be familiar with the physical and chemical properties that establish the hazardous characteristics of the materials used in a facility. The facility should have a documented process hazard analysis, and SH&E professionals should be familiar with the hazards identified in the study. A management of change program should be implemented. Also, SH&E professionals should be familiar with the requirements of the NFPA standards that apply to a facility. One obvious item to assess is housekeeping. Poor housekeeping may lead to accumulations of dust on machinery and building structural members. SH&E

professionals also should identify hidden areas that may not be obvious while standing at floor level. Other areas, such as spaces above drop ceilings and around ductwork junctions and gates, also should be inspected. Dust can accumulate on elevated building and equipment members. In the event of an initial ignition, the shock wave may shake this accumulation, creating another dust cloud and another potentially greater ignition that can shake even more dust from the elevated members, setting up a chain reaction. Process equipment should be designed for the operation in which it is used. Typically, initial installation of a process incorporates several features to help mitigate a fire or deflagration. These may include explosion vents on machines and/or buildings. It may be a fast-acting explosion suppression system. Gates and dampers may be installed inside of ductwork or equipment. Each device should be inspected and tested regularly, with documentation created to record and verify its condition. Conductive components should be grounded and bonded. Training is another important aspect of a dust hazard mitigation program. Operators should be trained on the equipment's operation and maintenance and emergency plans to follow. Initial as well as refresher training should be provided, and training records should be maintained.

11). Answer D:

The spring-loaded cover on a flammable liquid safety can allows excess vapor pressure to be vented through the cover. As vapor pressure builds up it unseats the spring cover and then closes automatically to again seal the container. Because of this potential for vapor release containers must not be stored or transported in confined spaces such as in the trunks of vehicles.

12) Answer A:

To determine the root cause, you need to determine the fire ignition source and the area of origin.

13) Answer D:

All of these factors govern the possibility of a dust explosion. Dust explosions usually occur as a series, the initial deflagration being rather small in volume but intense enough to jar dust from beams, ledges, etc. This causes larger concentrations to form and a second more destructive cycle will begin.

14) Answer C:

While the destructiveness of a dust explosion depends primarily on the rate of pressure rise, other factors are maximum pressure developed, the duration of the excess pressure, the degree of confinement of the explosion volume and the oxygen concentration.

15) Answer B:

This is the definition of a ground according to the NSC.

16) Answer A:

1926.152(d) "Fire control for flammable or combustible liquid storage."

- At least one portable fire extinguisher, having a rating of not less than 20-B units, shall be located outside of, but not more than 10 feet from, the door opening into any room used for storage of more than 60 gallons of flammable or combustible liquids.
- At least one portable fire extinguisher having a rating of not less than 20-B units shall be located not less than 25 feet, nor more than 75 feet, from any flammable liquid storage area located outside.

17) Answer B:

OSHAs position on labeling fire extinguishers is outlined in a letter from the Director of Compliance Programs dated May 15, 1993. " Subpart Z of the Hazard Communication Standard does apply to fire extinguishers. In terms of labeling requirements under the Hazard Communication Standard (HCS), only those fire extinguishers that contain hazardous chemicals, are required to be labeled. A compressed gas is defined as a physical hazard in the HCS. Therefore, those fire extinguishers containing compressed gas are required to be labeled under the HCS.

18)   Answer D:

In any emergency there is a possibility that the person (or persons) involved may not be able to escape under his/her own resources. Provisions must be made for rescue by other personnel, if the need should arise. Rescues may be attempted by:

- Persons familiar with the product and its operation, hazards, and emergency devices.
- Personnel familiar with the hazards in general but not the specific equipment.
- Untrained personnel who are unfamiliar with the product or the hazards involved but want to help.

19)   Answer A because

ICS is organized into three components—Incident Command, Command Staff, and General Staff positions. Incident Command can be comprised either of a single Incident Commander or a Unified Command. An example ICS organizational chart is shown

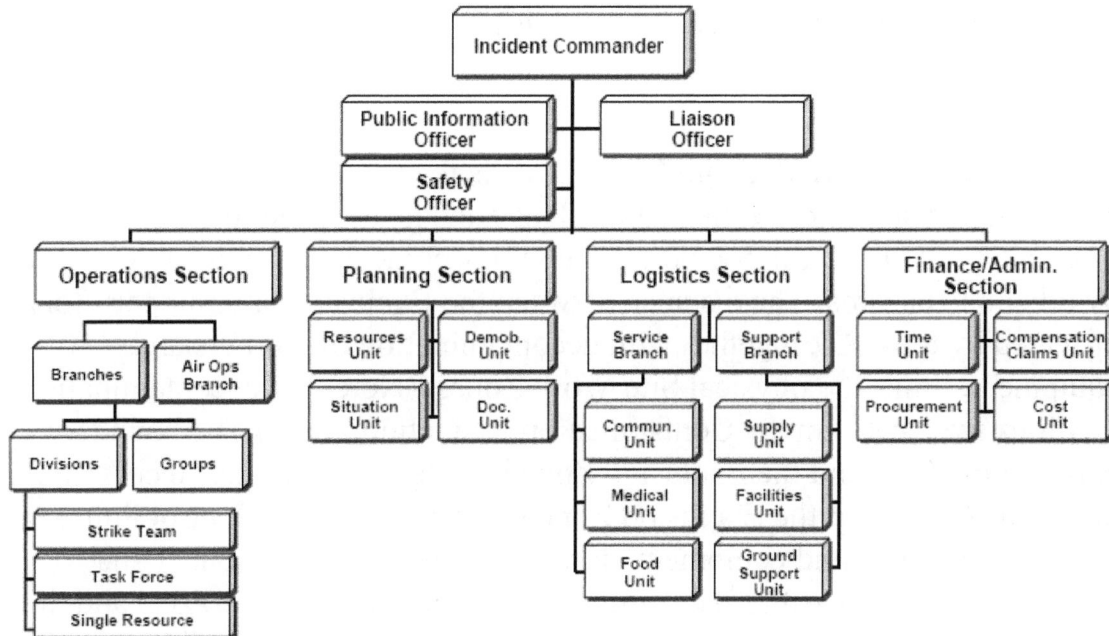

The Command Staff (CS) members perform incident-wide tasks and report directly to the IC. The three most common CS positions include:

- **Safety Officer** – responsible for the safe operations of all tasks performed on-site. The Safety Office has the essential authority to terminate any operations deemed to be unsafe, and even to override the authority of the IC to do so.
- **Public Information** Officer – the PIO is responsible for passing information regarding the incident to the public and to the media. Traditionally the PIO was responsible for press releases and public warning statements issued through the media. In recent years with the huge explosion of social media the PIO position has expanded greatly.
- **Liaison Officer** – this position is responsible for interacting and coordinating with other response entities not represented in the incident to provide their input on legal issues and resource availability.

20)   Answer A:

1926.152(c)(1) states "Storage of containers (not more than 60 gallons each) shall not exceed 1,100 gallons in any one pile or area. Piles or groups of containers shall be separated by a 5-foot clearance. Piles or groups of containers shall not be nearer than 20 feet to a building."

21).   Answer B:

The Contamination Reduction Zone (CRZ) is the transition area between the contaminated area and the clean area. This zone is designed to reduce the probability that the clean Support Zone will become contaminated or affected by other site hazards. The distance between the Exclusion and Support Zones provided by the CRZ, together with decontamination of workers and equipment, limits the physical Site Work Zones. (Note that decontamination facilities are located in the Contamination Reduction Zone.) The boundary between the CRZ and the Exclusion Zone is called the Hotline. Access into and out of the CRZ from the Exclusion Zone is through Access Control Points: one each for personnel and equipment entrance, one each for personnel and equipment exit, if feasible. The boundary between the Support Zone and the CRZ, called the Contamination Control Line, separates the possibly low contamination area from the clean Support Zone. Access to the CRZ from the Support Zone is through two Access Control Points if feasible: one each for personnel and equipment.

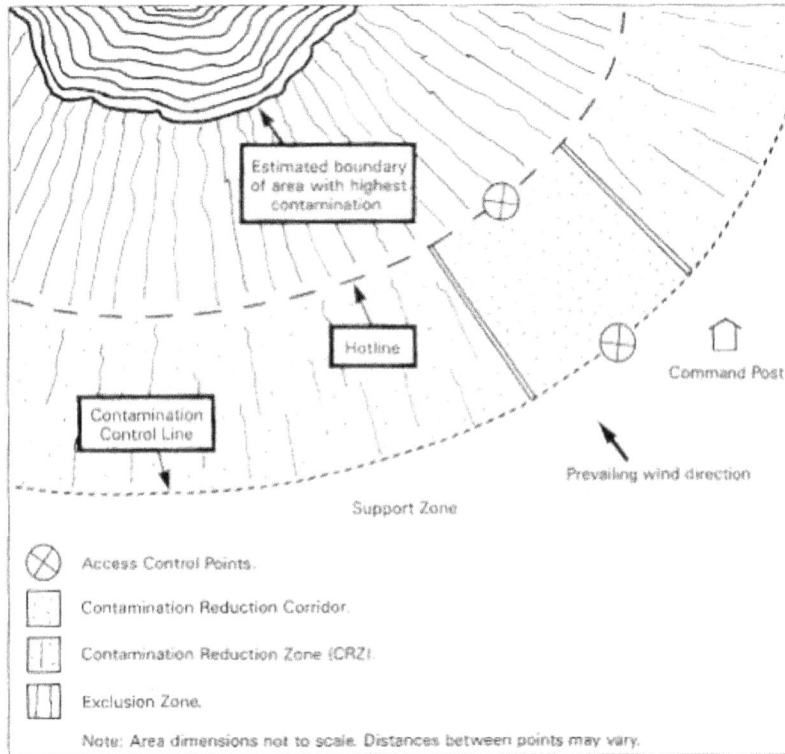

22). Answer C:

Most people know the class of fire extinguishers, but many do not pay attention to the shape associated with each class. Study the chart below and remember that 'dry chemical' is often associated with Class B or C, but 'dry powder' is associated with Class D.

Class A	Ordinary combustibles	Triangle
Class B	Flammable liquids	Square
Class C	Electrical	Circle
Class D	Combustible metals	Star
Class K	Vegetable oils/animal fats	Hexagon

23). Answer C:

GHS stands for the Globally Harmonized System which is the shortened version of the Globally Harmonized System of Classification and Labeling of Chemicals. The GHS was adopted by the United Nations (UN) in 2003 and the US incorporated it for full implementation by 2016. It includes criteria for the classification of health, physical and environmental hazards, as well as specifying what information should be included on labels of hazardous chemicals as well as safety data sheets. The United States was an active participant in the development of the GHS, and is a member of the UN bodies established to maintain and coordinate implementation of the system. The official text of the GHS can be found on the UN web page. For more information, see https://www.osha.gov/dsg/hazcom/global.html and https://www.osha.gov/dsg/hazcom/HCSFactsheet.html

24).   Answer B:

We assess that Coordination is the most important of the options given. The choice of MOST important could change based on the situation, prevailing conditions and the desired outcome. Because the question specifies this as an Incident Command situation, the scenario is most likely a disaster response where there will most likely be many organizations involved. Many of these organizations will not be under the 'command' of the incident commander. In addition, while communication is very important in any complex situation, simply communicating is not nearly as impactful as coordinating. Also, while cooperating is critical when cooperation is needed, it is often not needed whereas coordination will almost always produce opportunities for increased synergies.

25).   Answer A:

For communication to occur, you must have a sender that sends a message to a receiver. Typically, the sender will ask or watch for some feedback to ensure they have communicated. The sequence is sender-message-receiver-feedback.

Domain 2: Quiz 2 Questions

1). For fire protection, how does a building under construction compare to a completed building?

    A) Construction is significantly less at risk

    B) Construction is somewhat less at risk

    C) Construction is similarly at risk

    D) Construction is more at risk

2). Which of these is NOT a functional area of ICS?

    A) Planning,

    B) Logistics

    C) Supply

    D) Administration/Finance

3). How does a combustible gas meter display its readings?

    A) % of UEL

    B) % of PEL

    C) % of TLV

    D) % of LEL

4). What is this NOT a GHS pictogram for?

    A) Oxidizing gases, category 1

    B) Oxidizing liquids, categories 1, 2, 3

    C) Oxidizing solids, categories 1, 2, 3

    D) Organic peroxides, types B, C, D, E, F

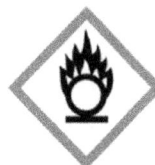

5). What is the GHS symbol for Explosives?

    A)

    B)

    C)

    D)

6). What is the GHS symbol for a Flammable?

A)

B)

C)

D)

7). What is the GHS symbol for Corrosive to Metals?

A)

B)

C)

D)

8). What is this NOT a GHS pictogram for?
   A) Acute toxicity (oral, dermal, inhalation), category 4
   B) Skin irritation/sensitization
   C) Narcotic effects
   D) Acute toxicity (oral, dermal, inhalation), categories 1, 2, 3

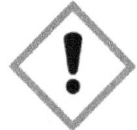

9). In emergency planning, what would a warning alarm be a form of?
   A) Preparedness & mitigation;
   B) Response
   C) Recovery
   D) Failure

10). Hazardous waste sites are often divided into many different zones as needed to meet operational and safety objectives. Which of these are NOT listed by OSHA as a frequently used zone for during decontamination operations: ·

A) Contamination Zone
B) Contamination Reduction Zone (CRZ)·
C) Support Zone
D) Exclusion Zone

11). Thirty-five gallons of flammable liquids are present on construction site, and not stored in a flammable storage cabinet. The **best** solution is to:

A) Move all of it off site, flammable liquids are not allowed on a construction site.
B) Advise supervisor to remove 10 gallons from the site, or place into an approved flammable storage cabinet.
C) Allow up to 60 gallons outside of an approved flammable storage cabinet on the site.
D) Advise workers to post a fire watch to monitor the job site for fires.

12). For emergency scene management, what are the proper sequence of actions?

A) Call EMS; secure the scene, care for injured, take photos, document evidence
B) Secure the scene, call EMS; care for injured, take photos, document evidence
C) Document evidence, call EMS; secure the scene, care for injured, take photos
D) Care for injured, secure the scene, Call EMS; take photos, document evidence

13). Which NFPA section is most related to building construction occupancy codes?

A) NFPA 101
B) NFPA 30
C) NFPA 10
D) NFPA 70

14). Which of these is NOT a functional area of ICS?
   A) Medical
   B) Planning
   C) Operations
   D) Logistics

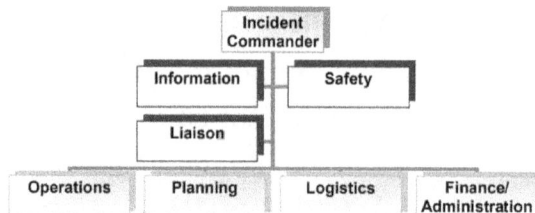

Copyright©2019 SPAN International Training, LLC

Domain 2: Quiz 2 Answers

1). Answer D:

Buildings under construction are considerably more at risk of a fire than completed buildings for several reasons, but the two most obvious are buildings under construction do not have the protections in place that finished buildings have and they typically have a concentration of construction materials and construction activities (welding, cutting, etc) present.

2). Answer C:

According to FEMA (Federal Emergency Management Agency), the functional areas of Incident Command System (ICS) Functional Areas of ICS ICS establishes the following five major functional areas for managing an incident:

Command – Provides leadership and establishes incident objectives as well as having overall responsibility for managing the incident;

Operations – Develops and oversees tactical operational activities needed to accomplish incident objectives;

Finance/Administration – Oversees all administrative and financial aspects of the incident including cost tracking, procurement, payments, compensation, etc. in support of objectives;

Planning – Coordinates planning, resource ordering and release, record keeping, mapping, technical expertise, and documentation necessary to accomplish objectives; and

Logistics – Oversees the development and use of infrastructures (facilities, transportation, supplies, communication, food, etc.) to support responders as they work towards accomplishing incident objectives.

There is no functional area called 'Supply'. Supply is part of the Logistics functional area.

3). Answer D:

Combustible gas meters display their readings in percent (%) of Lower Explosive Limit (LEL)

4). Answer D:

Know all the GHS pictograms and their associated hazards:

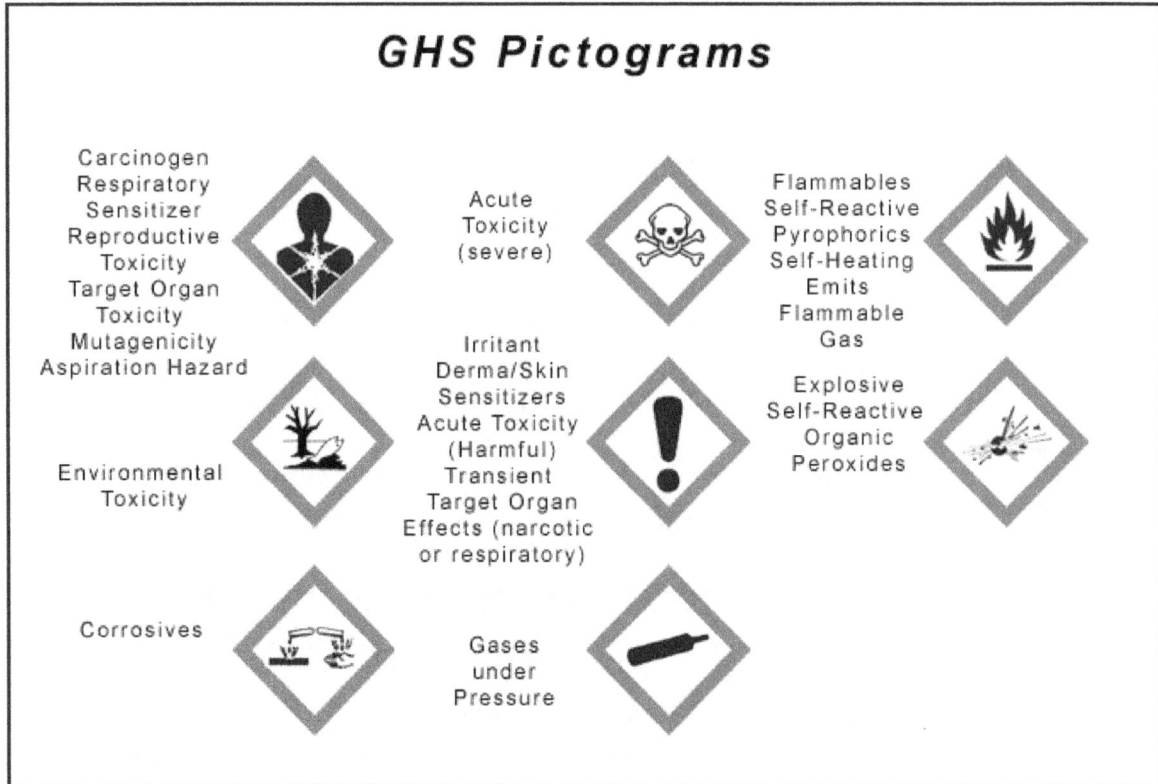

GHS Pictograms

Carcinogen
Respiratory
Sensitizer
Reproductive
Toxicity
Target Organ
Toxicity
Mutagenicity
Aspiration Hazard

Acute
Toxicity
(severe)

Flammables
Self-Reactive
Pyrophorics
Self-Heating
Emits
Flammable
Gas

Environmental
Toxicity

Irritant
Derma/Skin
Sensitizers
Acute Toxicity
(Harmful)
Transient
Target Organ
Effects (narcotic
or respiratory)

Explosive
Self-Reactive
Organic
Peroxides

Corrosives

Gases
under
Pressure

5). Answer A:

The pictogram for explosives is the warning diamond containing a representation of an element exploding.

6). Answer D:

The pictogram for a flammable is the warning diamond containing the representation of a fire.

7). Answer B:

The pictogram for a flammable is the warning diamond containing the representation of a fire.

8).   Answer D:

The warning diamond containing the explanation point is for acute toxicity (oral, dermal, inhalation), category 4, skin irritation/sensitization, or narcotic effects. Acute toxicity (oral, dermal, inhalation), categories 1, 2, 3 is the diamond containing a representation of the human torso with the expanding star in the chest. Acute toxicity category 5 is the diamond containing the skull and crossbones.

9).   Answer B:

During emergency planning often planners make use of some sort of alarm as a means to notify or alert people to certain conditions. This would be considered a form of response.

10).   Answer A:

OSHA's guidance document on hazardous waste states, "Hazardous waste sites should be divided into as many different zones as needed to meet operational and safety objectives. For illustration, this manual describes three frequently used zones:" ·

- Exclusion Zone, the contaminated area. ·
- Contamination Reduction Zone (CRZ), the area where decontamination takes place. ·
- Support Zone, the uncontaminated area where workers should not be exposed to hazardous conditions.

https://www.osha.gov/Publications/complinks/OSHG-HazWaste/9-10.pdf

11).   Answer B:

1926.152(b)(1) states "No more than 25 gallons of flammable liquids shall be stored in a room outside of an approved storage cabinet." While removing 10 gallons to another area is not the best course of action, it is an acceptable course of action in this case.

12).   Answer A:

In any emergency situation, the first action should always be sending for assistance of some sort (sounding the alarm, calling out, etc.). Many times, first responders are injured because they get tunnel vision on the injured and do not make sure it is safe to approach so the second action must be to secure the scene. Next, we should provide care to injured within our abilities. Next, we begin to preserve evidence by taking photos and other documentation in order to investigate and prevent recurrence.

13).   Answer A:

NFPA 101 is the **Life Safety Code** is the NFPA most concerned with occupancy. NFPA 10 covers portable fire extinguishers. NFPA 30 is the **Flammable and Combustible Liquids Code**. NFPA 70 is the **National Electric Code (NEC)**.

14).   Answer A:

According to FEMA (Federal Emergency Management Agency), the functional areas of Incident Command System (ICS) Functional Areas of ICS establishes the following five major functional areas for managing an incident:

Command – Provides leadership and establishes incident objectives as well as having overall responsibility for managing the incident;

Operations – Develops and oversees tactical operational activities needed to accomplish incident objectives;

Finance/Administration – Oversees all administrative and financial aspects of the incident including cost tracking, procurement, payments, compensation, etc. in support of objectives;

Planning – Coordinates planning, resource ordering and release, record keeping, mapping, technical expertise, and documentation necessary to accomplish objectives; and

Logistics – Oversees the development and use of infrastructures (facilities, transportation, supplies, communication, food, etc.) to support responders as they work towards accomplishing incident objectives.

There is no functional area called 'Medical.

Domain 3: Safety Program Development and Implementation

Domain 3 *Safety Program Development and Implementation* • 17.1%

Knowledge of:

12. Applicable health and safety standards and best practices (e.g., health, safety, construction, and environmental)
13. Common components of site-specific safety plans
14. Worksite assessment or audit processes
15. Roles, responsibilities, and lines of authority as they relate to safety management
16. Recommended equipment inspection records or logs
17. Basic risk management concepts (e.g., public safety, builder's risk and liabilities, general liability)
18. General/basic construction site conditions that could potentially impact safety
19. Data gathering techniques and procedures used in incident investigations
20. Techniques for determining the root cause of accidents or incidents
21. Post-incident/accident reporting and follow-up procedures
22. Documentation requirements of occupational injuries and illnesses

Skill to:

5. Identify which health and safety programs (e.g., fall protection, ladders, respiratory) are relevant to site-specific safety plan
6. Apply relevant standards to worksite conditions
7. Identify trends related to incidents and accidents
8. Evaluate construction means and methods and their impact on safety

Occupational Health and Safety Management Systems

A management system is a set of interrelated elements used to establish policy and objectives and implement strategies to achieve those objectives. A management system includes organizational structure, planning activities, responsibilities, practices, procedures, processes, and resources. The conventional model for a management framework that follows a logical progression of activities aimed at improving the performance of the organization is the "Plan, Do, Check, Act" or PDCA cycle.

An organization may choose to implement a management system for many reasons, such as enhancing business performance through the following:

- Developing a management structure that is effective and responsive to the organization's needs
- Making operational improvements
- Changing the operational culture
- Marketing opportunities and improving public image
- Improving relationships with regulators
- Enhancing the ability to meet regulatory requirements and reduced costs from penalties
- Providing for greater employee involvement, awareness and commitment to performance, and improving morale
- Complying with a client's requirements

Occupational Health & Safety Management Systems (OHSMS's) consist of six "core elements". Each core element is important and necessary to ensure the success of the overall system. All the elements are interrelated and interdependent. The core elements are:

1). Management Leadership
2). Employee Participation
3). Hazard Identification and Assessment
4). Hazard Prevention and Control
5). Education and Training
6). System Evaluation and Continuous Improvement

A summary of the core elements of an effective occupational health and safety management systems (OHSMS) include:

Management Leadership
• Establish clear safety and health objectives for the OHSMS and operationally define the actions needed to achieve those objectives.
• Designate one or more individuals with overall responsibility for implementing and maintaining the OHSMS.
• Provide sufficient resources to ensure effective OHSMS implementation.

Employee [Worker] Participation
• Consult with employees in developing and implementing the system and involve them in updating and evaluating the OHSMS.
• Include employees in workplace inspections, incident investigations, and solutions.
• Encourage employees to report concerns, such as hazards, injuries, illnesses and near misses.

Hazard Identification and Risk Assessment
• Identify, assess and document workplace hazards with activities such as soliciting input from workers, inspecting the workplace and reviewing available information on hazards and risks.
• Investigate incidents that in involve both injuries and illnesses and near misses to identify hazards that may have caused them. The purpose is prevention.
• Inform employees of the hazards and risks in the workplace.

The core elements of an effective occupational health and safety management systems (OHSMS) continued:

Hazard Prevention and Control
• Establish and implement a plan to prioritize and control hazards and risks identified in the workplace.
• Provide both interim and permanent controls that reduce the risk of exposure to hazards and protect employees.
• Verify that all control measures are implemented and are effective.
• Discuss the hazard control plan with affected employees.

Education and Training

• Provide education and training to employees in a language and vocabulary they can understand to ensure that they know:
    o Procedures for reporting injuries, illnesses and safety and health concerns.
    o How to recognize hazards.
    o Ways to eliminate, control or reduce hazards.
    o Elements of the program.
    o How to participate in the program.

• Conduct refresher education and training programs periodically.

System Evaluation and Continuous Improvement
• Conduct a periodic review of the safety management system to determine if it has been implemented as designed and is making progress towards achieving its goals.
• Modify the program, as necessary, to correct deficiencies.
• Continuously look for ways to improve the OHSMS.

Employee Participation

Employee involvement provides the means through which workers develop and express their own commitment to safety and health, for both themselves and their fellow workers. It is also key to getting accurate risk assessments, workers closest to the operations usually have the best knowledge of the methods, tasks, breakdowns and problems. The findings and lessons arising from all evaluation and corrective action activities become part of the information that feeds back to the employee participation process

Employees should be involved:

- They are the persons most in contact with potential safety and health hazards. They have a vested interest in effective protection systems.
- Group decisions have the advantage of the group's wider range of experience.
- Employees are more likely to support and use programs in which they have input.
- Employees who are encouraged to offer their ideas and whose contributions are taken seriously are more satisfied and productive on the job.

Examples of employee participation include:

Participating on joint labor-management committees and other advisory or specific purpose committees.

- Conducting site inspections.
- Analyzing routine hazards in each step of a job or process, and preparing safe work practices or controls to eliminate or reduce exposure.
- Developing and revising the site safety and health rules.
- Training both current and newly hired employees.
- Providing programs and presentations at safety and health meetings.
- Conducting accident/incident investigations.
- Reporting hazards.
- Fixing hazards within your control.
- Supporting your fellow workers by providing feedback on risks and assisting them in eliminating hazards.
- Participating in accident/incident investigations.
- Performing a pre-use or change analysis for new equipment or processes in order to identify hazards up front before use.

Domain 3: Quiz 1 Questions

1). A major construction project management team implemented a series of toolbox safety meetings held at the beginning of each shift; housekeeping initiatives; barricade performance for elevated areas; and management walk thru audits to demonstrate leadership and commitment. These activities are most generally categorized as:

    A) Union organizing inhibitors.
    B) Leading indicators.
    C) Lagging indicators.
    D) Cost indicators.

2). The technique of system safety analysis can be applied to which of the following?

    A) Generally, only on the most complex of processes or systems.
    B) Very simple systems with only a single component.
    C) Any system that has interacting components.
    D) Any system only after some loss has occurred.

3). Which of the following descriptions best fits the intent referring to a "Competent Person"?

    A) The person required at confined space, and hoisting & rigging, and excavation & trenching job sites.
    B) The supervisor with the ability of identifying existing and future hazards on the job site and who reports directly to the person who has responsible charge of the operation.
    C) The person who has the authority to shut down the operation anytime the risk analysis indicates that a moderate or greater hazard is reasonably expected to cause injury to workers.
    D) The person capable of identifying hazards in the working conditions and authorized to act corrective measures to control.

4). Which of the following is not a specific duty of a competent person during underground construction operations?

    A) Air monitoring.
    B) Inspection of all drilling equipment prior to each use.
    C) Inspection of all hauling equipment prior to each shift.
    D) Inspection of barricades used to seal off unused headings.

5). The simplest and most effective way to display data to get an instant picture is the use of the?
    A) Line chart.
    B) Bar chart.
    C) Pie chart.
    D) Area chart.

6). The OSHA construction standards establish certain qualifications for blasters. Which of the following is not included in those qualifications?
    A) Possession of a state blasters license.
    B) Knowledge and competency in the use of each type of blasting method to be used on the job.
    C) Must be able to read and write.
    D) Good physical condition.

7). As described in *ANSI/ASSE* Z10-2012, for an organization's occupational health and safety management system to succeed, top management leadership and which of the following is most critical?
    A) Supervisor accountability.
    B) Employee participation.
    C) OHS written policy.
    D) Sustainable safety observation program.

8). At least ___ designated person(s) shall be on duty above ground whenever any employee is working underground and shall be responsible for securing immediate aid and keeping an accurate count of employees underground in case of emergency.
    A) None.
    B) One.
    C) Two.
    D) Depends on the size of the underground operation.

9). Which of the following is considered to be the primary reason for accident investigation for Safety and Health reasons?
    A) To determine the facts surrounding the event.
    B) To establish who or what was at fault.
    C) To determine the obvious cause factors.
    D) To establish a baseline for further analysis.

10). Which of the following is not generally included when determining the facts surrounding an incident?
   A) Injury classifications
   B) Hazardous Condition Classification
   C) Workers Compensation Rating
   D) Unsafe Acts

11). The primary reason safety professionals perform accident investigation is to:
   A) Discipline rule violators
   B) Provide OSHA and the country with valid information
   C) Satisfy the insurance carrier
   D) Determine causal conditions

12). Sources of information that might be used for injury accident analysis include all of the following except:
   A) First-Aid Reports
   B) Insurance rate table
   C) First report of injury form
   D) Supervisor accident investigation

13). The use of a registered Professional Engineer (P.E.) to ensure the safety of complicated, unusual or high-risk structures. Which of the following would not require the services of a registered professional engineer?
   A) To determine if an excavation's distance from buildings could disrupt the foundation.
   B) To design frame scaffolds more than 125 feet in height
   C) To design sloping and benching plans for excavations in type "C" soil deeper than 16 feet
   D) To design personnel hoists in bridge tower construction

14). Accident costs are generally divided into two areas. What are these two areas?
   A) Budgeted and Non-Budgeted
   B) Insured and Uninsured
   C) Direct and Indirect
   D) Direct and Uninsured

15). Which of the following typically does most of the accident investigations within the industrial community?
   A) Supervisor
   B) Manager
   C) Chief Executive Officer
   D) Safety Engineer

16). Which of the following is not a primary reason safety professionals' perform accident investigation?
   A) To prevent reoccurrence of similar events
   B) To assemble mishap data to search for trends
   C) To determine who or what was at fault
   D) To gather facts and opinions

17). In an active mishap prevention program, who should investigate a serious or fatal accident?
   A) A senior management official
   B) The safety engineers
   C) The supervisor
   D) The insurance investigator

18). Accident investigation is done for many reasons. Often several accident investigators will be at the scene of an accident at the same time. Which of the following is the least important task with respect to the CHSTs accident investigation responsibilities?
   A) Getting to the scene before anybody else
   B) Preventing the second accident
   C) Preserving evidence
   D) Taking care of, or transporting the injured

19). From most important to least important, which of the following indicates the correct order of actions to be taken by an accident investigator?
   A) 1,2,3,4   1.   Arrive safely
   B) 1,3,2,4   2.   Care for the injured
   C) 1,4,2,3   3.   Size-up the situation
   D) 1,2,4,3   4.   Protect property

20). When doing accident investigation, the interviewing of witnesses is often required to determine facts relative to the event and access to the accident scene is not an option. Which of the following choices offers the best place to conduct interviews for safety investigations?

    A) A secure board room equipped with sound recording devices
    B) In your office with the door shut
    C) At the employees work area
    D) In a neutral private conference room

21). Which of the following best answers the question, when should accident investigation begin?

    A) Within 48 hours of the time the accident scene is secured, that is, emergency services has left the site
    B) Immediately - the sooner the better
    C) As soon as possible, realizing that protection of the injured and prevention of a second accident will take precedence
    D) As soon as all legal notifications have been made and the scene secured against destruction of evidence

22). Which of the following is not a required element in the OSHA mandated respirator program?

    A) Training in the use of respirators
    B) All rescue respirators must be cleaned immediately after use
    C) Respirators must be inspected at regular intervals
    D) Respirators must not be used by more than one employee

23). Who has the responsibility to determine chemical health effects?

    A) All employees have this right
    B) Unionized employees have this right
    C) The employer is legally obligated to make this determination
    D) The manufacturer or importer of the chemical

24). On multi-employer worksites implementation of the Hazard Communication Program poses some additional concerns. If the general contractor handles or uses hazardous chemicals in such a manner that sub-contract employees working on the site may be exposed then the general contractor is required do which of the following?
   A) Instruct the sub to retrain all their employees on the Hazard Communication Standard due to a new hazard in the workplace
   B) Provide the sub with a SDS or notify the sub where the SDSs are centrally located for each hazardous material they may be exposed to while working on site
   C) Call the manufacturer and have them send a new SDS to the sub-contractor for each hazardous material they may be exposed to while working on site
   D) Provide training on the Hazard Communication Standard to all employees of the sub-contractor detailing the differences in the procedures of the two different companies

25). While reviewing the plans for a sewer line project to be performed by a sub-contractor you are puzzled by the definition of a "trench excavation" used throughout the document. Which of the following is the best definition of a trench excavation?
   A) A hole deeper than wide
   B) Any excavation less than 20 feet in depth that is longer than it is wide
   C) An excavation where the dimension "b" is greater than the dimension "a" as long as "a" is less than two times "b"
   D) A narrow excavation where the depth is greater than the width but not wider than 15 feet.

Domain 3: Quiz 1 Answers

1) Answer B:

According to authors Marlowe and Skrabak (2007), the selection of leading indicators is largely judgmental and only time will tell whether the indicators selected are the right ones. It seems logical to suggest that the leading indicators selected should relate directly to opportunities to reduce risk by improving those safety management processes that analysis indicates need improvement, on a prioritized basis. In safety-related literature, the most commonly identified lagging indicators are accidents and cost trends, and sometimes near misses. Toolbox safety meetings held at the beginning of each shift; housekeeping; barricade performance for elevated areas; and management walking around to show leadership and commitment are generally considered examples of leading indicators.

2) Answer C:

The discipline of system safety can be applied to almost any system that has interacting components. It is an application of systematic and forward looking techniques to identify and control hazards. The discipline is most effective if it begins within the conceptual phases of project development and should continue throughout the entire life of the project or product.

3) Answer D:

OSHA defines a competent person as "one who is capable of identifying existing and predictable hazards in the surroundings or working conditions which are unsanitary, hazardous, or dangerous to employees, and who has authorization to take prompt corrective measures to eliminate them". Additionally, the competent person should be a person who has extensive knowledge/experience in a particular activity or job function.

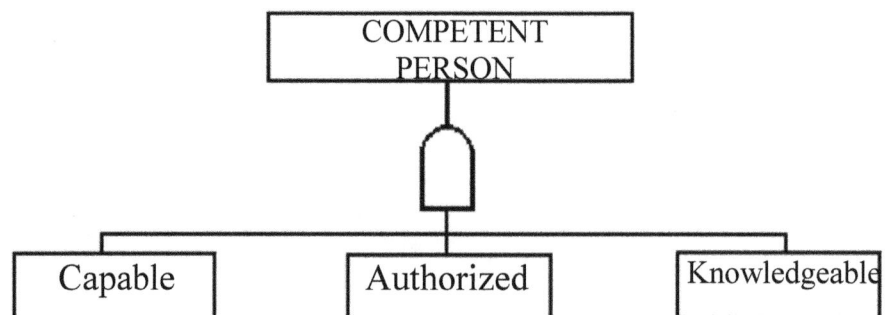

The result is a system fed by an "and" gate. The competent person must be capable "and" authorized "and" knowledgeable. Failure of any one of the elements results in a failure of the entire system.

4)   Answer D:

Underground construction covers the construction of underground tunnels, shafts, chambers and cut-and-cover excavations. The regulation establishes a "competent person" as the responsible party for various inspection and oversight operations in the underground environment. In accordance with OSHA 1926.800 a competent person is responsible for:
- Air monitoring
- Testing the atmosphere for flammable limits before restoring power and equipment and before returning to work after a ventilation system has been shut down due to hazardous levels of flammable gas or methane
- Inspection of the work area for ground stability
- Inspection of all drilling equipment prior to each use
- Inspection of all hauling equipment before each shift
- Visually checking all hoisting machinery, equipment, anchorages, and rope at the beginning of each shift and during hoisting if necessary

The inspection of barricaded headings is not specifically covered in the OSHA directives.

5)   Answer B:

The recommended use of the bar chart is to illustrate comparisons of volume over time

6)   Answer A:

Federal OSHA does not specifically require a state blasters license, although the state you are operating in may very well have such a requirement. OSHA does require that a blaster:

- Be able to understand and give written and oral orders
- Shall be in good physical condition and not be addicted to narcotics, intoxicants, or similar types of drugs
- Shall be qualified, by reason of training, knowledge, or experience, in the field of transporting, storing, handling, and use of explosives, and have a working knowledge of State and local laws and regulations which pertain to explosives

7)   Answer B:

According to *ANSI/ASSE Z10-2012*, top management leadership and employee participation are the main divisions in the scope of this standard.

8)   Answer B:

1926.800(g)(3) Designated person: At least one designated person shall be on duty above ground whenever any employee is working underground. This designated person shall be responsible for securing immediate aid and keeping an accurate count of employees underground in case of emergency. The designated person must not be so busy that the counting function is encumbered.

9)   Answer A:

According to the National Safety Council accident investigation should be conducted to provide the facts, if fault-finding is attempted the investigation may cause more harm than good. Mishap investigation is conducted to determine both obvious and hidden cause factors. It does tend to serve as the baseline for further analysis but selection "A" is the *primary* reason for investigation.

10) Answer C:

ANSI Z16.2 is designed to provide a standardized method of recording certain accident facts. ANSI Z16.2 does not include any provisions for recording workers compensation information. The classifications that are included are:
- Nature of Injury
- Part of Body Affected
- Source of Injury
- Accident Type
- Hazardous Condition
- Agency of Accident
- Agency of Accident Part
- Unsafe Act

11) Answer D:

Accidents or mishaps are investigated by safety and health professionals to determine the root cause factors and to prevent future occurrences of the same type by implementing appropriate corrective actions. This goal must be kept in mind throughout the investigation process. Many times, other investigations are being conducted for other reasons, for example, security, personnel or possibly even the legal staff may be interested in facts surrounding any unusual event. These investigations usually are searching for discipline, reimbursement, protection from liability, litigation or the assessment of blame. It is not uncommon for the safety professional to be drawn into these investigations because of their investigative skills and in-depth knowledge of the job site. However, it is imperative that accident prevention investigations be separated from discipline investigations if one is to find the true cause factors. Firing the person who had the accident, rarely will prevent the next one.

12) Answer B:

The insurance rate table provides little or no useful information for analysis of accidents since it is most often based on past experience.

13) Answer C:

There is continuing controversy over the use of the terms registered professional engineer, professional engineer, a competent engineer etc. within the OSHA directives. OSHA has promised standardization in the near future for the "Professional Engineer" requirement and a raft of other misused or undefined terms i.e.; certified, competent, qualified, highly qualified, registered etc. However, according to the current OSHA standards selection "A" is correct. 1926.651 requires a P.E. determine if an excavation will affect adjacent structures. Selection "B" is also correct 1926.451(d)(9) requires the services of a P.E. in designing frame scaffolds in excess of 125 ft in height. Selection "C" is not correct.

The P.E. is only required to be involved if the excavation is at a depth of 20 feet or greater. Selection "D" is correct and can be found at 1926.552(c)(17)(i).

14) Answer C:

Accident costs have for many years been divided into direct and indirect costs. Direct costs are those costs directly and often immediately associated with the accident such as: transportation of the injured, medical services, days lost from work etc. Indirect costs would include: lost production, replacement of the injured worker, costs of training a replacement etc. The indirect costs associated with accidents rarely consider the effects of a mishap on family members.

15) Answer A:

The supervisor is the prime investigator in most industrial accidents. They are closest to the action, they are most familiar with the environment and the resultant interactions and stresses that occur. Supervisors are positioned in exactly the right position to provide valuable insight into the process, which caused the accident, and to recommend corrective action to remedy the problem. Strangely enough, these are also the very same reasons the supervisor is not the correct person to do an in-depth investigation that will produce long lasting corrective actions. The supervisor is personally involved in the operation. He or she probably has friends among the workers. The credibility of the supervisor's position is on the line during any accident investigation. Can the supervisor honestly conduct an investigation that will in the final analysis point out deficiencies in management or supervision? Can they take off the company hat and become an impartial critic of the system, of themselves? Often the answer to this question is a resounding no! However, in spite of these obvious conflicts, the job of routine accident investigation still falls on the supervisors more often than not in the industrial environment.

16)   Answer C:

Accident investigation should be a fact-finding exercise designed to prevent occurrence of the same or similar events. The determination of fault should be left up to someone else. If safety investigations become fault finding investigations, they lose the ability to be objective and to find long lasting solutions to managerial or technical deficiencies.

17)   Answer A:

Senior management should investigate:
- Fatal accidents
- Accidents with large losses or the potential for large losses
- Mishaps that result or could result in adverse public reaction

Lower levels of supervision and the safety director/engineer should also be involved in these investigations. The safety engineer should act as the company resident expert in mishap investigation procedures and techniques offering advice and possibly training to other members of the investigation team. Most progressive companies also provide a standardized accident investigation "system" to be used on all important or large mishap investigations. The systems are varied and take many forms. They may be as simple as a checklist of items to be examined with a cause and effect report format or an extensive system that details the entire investigative effort from membership to analysis to formal reporting with corporate presentations.

18)   Answer A:

There is no doubt that an investigator's first tasking is to get to the scene safely. Everyone is in a hurry to get to the scene of the accident, but you cannot render assistance or perform an adequate investigation if you do not arrive safely. The job of a health and safety professional cannot start until the scene is secured, meaning that the injured are taken care of and the scene itself is made safe. If you arrive earlier than this you run the risk of becoming part of the emergency services effort which tends to make you part of the response rather than part of the investigative team. There are exceptions, such as in the case of the safety engineer who is part of the rescue or re-entry team, but in most cases the advice is solid.

19)   Answer B:

It is generally accepted within the health and safety community that the order of sequence for accident investigation should be:
- Arrive safely

You cannot do anyone any good if you are involved in an accident yourself racing to the scene of a tragedy. Once on the scene, **isolate it and control the access** to prevent further mishaps.
- Size up

The professional fire service uses the term "size-up" to indicate the time spent observing and analyzing the event. The same tactic should be used by investigators to determine what evidence must be protected, who is involved, who is on the scene, is the site now safe or is another mishap about to occur etc. Experience will allow you to accomplish this task very fast.
- Care for injured

If necessary the investigator should help injured and protect property. However, the investigators job is to gather facts not provide emergency service. Generally this job is best left to others. It is fine to render aid if you are needed but don't get in the way of the professionals.
- Protect property

Prevention of the second accident is an important aspect of the accident investigators job. Because of their observation skills and training safety professionals can often spot unsafe conditions that others involved in the emergency will not see. You must above all else not allow an accident to escalate into a disaster.

20)   Answer D:

This is a difficult question because the best place to do interviews changes with conditions. The investigator needs to make sure the witness feels at ease during the interview, which may mean conducting the interview at a location where the witness feels comfortable. However, the place where the interview takes place must also provide privacy. Often the ideal place to interview witnesses is at the accident scene itself. This allows the witness a visual reference, fosters understanding and aids memory. Witnesses should always be interviewed individually so that you won't get agreement from the group.

21)   Answer C:

Prompt investigation of the accident scene including interviewing witnesses is of utmost importance, however protection of the injured and prevention of a second accident must come first.

22)   Answer D:

Respirators may be used by more than one worker, however they must be cleaned and disinfected before use by another employee. They cannot simply be passed from person to person on a job site. All of the other selections are correct. Respirator users must be trained in the use and limitations of the apparatus. Respirators must be inspected at regular intervals and rescue equipment must be cleaned immediately after use so that the equipment is available should another emergency arise.

23)   Answer D:

OSHA states "Chemical manufacturers and importers shall evaluate chemicals produced in their workplaces or imported by them to determine if they are hazardous. Employers are not required to evaluate chemicals unless they choose not to rely on the evaluation performed by the chemical manufacturer or importer for the chemical to satisfy this requirement".

24)   Answer B:

The following information has been extracted and paraphrased from 29 CFR 1926.59. The Hazard Communication Program on multi-employer worksites where the employers produce, use, or store hazardous chemicals in such a way that other employers may be exposed shall develop a program that includes the following:
- The methods the employer will use to provide the other employers with a copy of the MSDS, or make it available at a central location on the worksite.
- The methods the employer will use to inform the other employers of any precautionary measures that need to be taken to protect employees during the workplace's normal operating conditions and in foreseeable emergencies.

- The methods the employer will use to inform the other employers of the labeling system used in the workplace.

25)   Answer D:

OSHA at 1926.650 defines a trench or trench excavation as "...a narrow excavation (in relation to its length) made below the surface of the ground. In general, the depth is greater than the width, but the width of a trench (measured at the bottom) is not greater than 15 feet. If forms or other structures are installed or constructed in an excavation so as to reduce the dimension measured from the forms or structure to the side of the excavation to 15 feet or less (measured at the bottom of the excavation), the excavation is also considered to be a trench.

Domain 3: Quiz 2 Questions

1). During the review of job plans, you notice that the contractor has a very broad use of the term "competent person". Which of the following best defines a "Competent Person"?

    A) The person required at confined space, and hoisting & rigging, and excavation & trenching job sites

    B) The supervisor with the ability of identifying existing and future hazards on the job site and who reports directly to the person who has responsible charge of the operation

    C) The person who has the authority to shut down the operation anytime the risk analysis indicates that a moderate or greater hazard is reasonably expected to cause injury to workers

    D) The person who is capable of identifying existing and predictable hazards in the surroundings or working conditions which are unsanitary, hazardous, or dangerous to employees, and who has authorization to take prompt corrective measures to eliminate them

2). On a multi-employer worksite, the general contractor has agreed to act as an intermediary for storage of the SDSs for the entire site. An OSHA inspector found several containers of hazardous chemicals without a label or SDS in some sub-contractors' trailer. A short investigation by the Compliance Officer revealed that the sub-contractor failed to notify the general he had the hazardous materials. Who would be cited for this violation?

    A) The sub-contractor

    B) The general contractor

    C) The owner

    D) Both general and sub-contractor

3). While reviewing a bid proposal from a sub-contractor for a lengthy construction job on a large site, the contractor has proposed several options for developing and complying with safety and health procedures. Which of the following will produce the most effective safety and health interface?

    A) The sub-contractor should develop their own procedures and follow them to the letter

    B) The sub-contractor should use the general contractor's procedures to provide site standardization

    C) The sub-contractor should follow all the OSHA rules and thus will not need procedures

    D) The sub-contractor should develop their own procedures with assistance from the general contractor

4). Which of the following are used to adjust Worker's Compensation Insurance Rates?

    A) Experience Modification Rate

    B) Incident Rate

    C) Worker's Compensation Mod Rate

    D) Accident Rate

5). An audit of safety and health program management has revealed that the program has failed to accomplish the stated objective of accident prevention. Accident rates are very poor, as is morale and discipline. Supervisors openly defy management authority and varying standards exist through the company. Which of the following offers the best explanation for the failure of safety program management?

    A) Failure of the safety director to establish an effective program

    B) Failure of top management to support the accident prevention effort

    C) Failure of management at all levels to manage, lead and direct the workforce

    D) Failure of procedures to identify the correct and safe methods for job accomplishment

6). Many injuries on the construction site are caused by material handling accidents. Several techniques have proven to be effective in preventing accidents of this type. Which of the following would be the least effective single element in the prevention of materials handling mishaps?
  A) Training
  B) Stringent physical requirements
  C) Job placement
  D) Job descriptions

7). Permit required confined spaces requires all of the following on a permit except?
  A) The permit space to be entered
  B) The purpose of the entry
  C) The name of the CEO or President
  D) The date and the authorized duration of the entry permit

8). The primary reason safety professionals perform accident investigation is to determine causal conditions. The responsibility for correcting the accident causes is the:
  A) Supervisor
  B) Safety Administrator
  C) Senior Safety Engineer
  D) Plant Manager

9). All of the following are valid reasons for accident (mishap) investigation except?
  A) Prevent reoccurrence of similar events
  B) Establish casual factors
  C) Provide vehicle for discipline
  D) Provide data for trend analysis

10). Which of the following is the definition of the management term "span of control"?
  A) The breadth of a manager's expertise
  B) The number of subordinates a manager can supervise
  C) The number of projects a manager can supervise
  D) The number of organizations a manager can supervise

11). Process Safety Management of Highly Hazardous Materials requires employers to establish a compliance audit capability. The standard calls for employers to certify that they have evaluated compliance with process safety requirements at least every _____ years.
    A) Two years
    B) Three years
    C) Four years
    D) Five years

12). Which is the most appropriate measurement of individual safety performance?
    A) Recognize workers for reporting hazards and correcting them
    B) Group performing thus far without injuries
    C) No safety discipline in the past year
    D) Crew completes entire job without a recordable injury

13). Are safety data sheets (SDSs) required for hazardous waste?
    A) No, SDSs are only required for hazardous chemicals
    B) Yes, SDSs are required for all hazardous substances
    C) No, unless generated in a threshold quantity
    D) Yes, if generated by a non-governmental agency

14). When it is not possible to interview people at the accident site, what is the next best place to interview a witness?
    A) Break room
    B) Conference room
    C) Your office
    D) Supervisors office

15). The Z-10 committee of SH&E professionals and stakeholders authored a consensus standard incorporating lessons learned and best practices in Occupational Safety and Health Management. Which of the following is not one of the major provisions of the standard?
    A) applying a prescribed hierarchy of controls to achieve acceptable levels of risk levels
    B) design reviews
    C) regulatory compliance
    D) management of change systems

16). Safety and Health Management Systems such as BSI 18001 series and ANSI/ASSE Z10 are built on established principles and process. Which of the following accurately describes the systems process?
   A) Act-Do-Plan-Check
   B) Plan-Do-Check-Act
   C) Plan-Act-Do-Check
   D) Check-Plan-Do-Act

17). Accident investigation is done for many reasons. Often several accident investigators will be at the scene of an accident at the same time. Which of the following is the most important task with respect to the CHST's accident investigation responsibilities?
   A) Getting to the scene before anybody else
   B) Preventing the second accident
   C) Preserving evidence
   D) Taking care of, or transporting the injured

18). Pareto charts are used to answer all of the following questions except?
   A) What are the largest issues facing our team or business?
   B) What 20% of sources are causing 80% of the problems (80/20 Rule)?
   C) Where should we focus our efforts to achieve the greatest improvements?
   D) Where are the indirect costs of incidents?

19). Which of the following are examples of indirect costs of an incident?
   A) Drug testing and ambulance service
   B) Incident review and process delays
   C) Medical treatment supplies and medical related treatment
   D) Job accommodations and new equipment

20). When removing shoring from a trench, it should be removed in which sequence?
   A) top to bottom
   B) bottom to top
   C) middle down, then middle up
   D) any sequence determined best by the supervisor

21). When the height of a supported scaffold (a scaffold with legs) is more than _____ its narrowest base dimension, it must be tied to a structure.
   A) 2 times
   B) 3 times
   C) 4 times
   D) 6 times

22). Which if the following is **true** about the use of wooden ladders?
   A) Can be used around electrical lines
   B) Should not be painted with an opaque finish
   C) Can be used if defects are identified
   D) The minimum clearance between fixed ladder rungs shall be 6 inches

23). The **best** location for a worker to tie-off to an anchor point is:
   A) Below the work level
   B) At or above the work level
   C) At or below the work level
   D) Above the work level

24). The **best** way to inspect chains during a semi-annual inspection is to:
   A) Check links with a caliper and compare at least 10 links
   B) Check for cracks in end links
   C) Compare twist on end sections
   D) Perform a detailed link-by-link inspection of entire chain

25). The standard requires that all materials stored in tiers be stacked, racked, blocked, interlocked, or otherwise secured to prevent sliding, falling or collapse. Which of the following statements would be correct concerning the stacking of bricks?
   A) Bricks must not be stacked over 8 feet in height
   B) Bricks must not be stacked over 6 feet in height
   C) Bricks stacks must be tapered back 1½ inches in every foot of height above the 3-foot level
   D) Bricks stacks must be tapered back 2 inches in every foot of height above the 4-foot level

Domain 3: Quiz 2 Answers

1). Answer D:

OSHA defines a competent person as "one who is capable of identifying existing and predictable hazards in the surroundings or working conditions which are unsanitary, hazardous, or dangerous to employees, and who has authorization to take prompt corrective measures to eliminate them". Additionally, the competent person should be a person who has extensive knowledge/experience in a particular activity or job function.

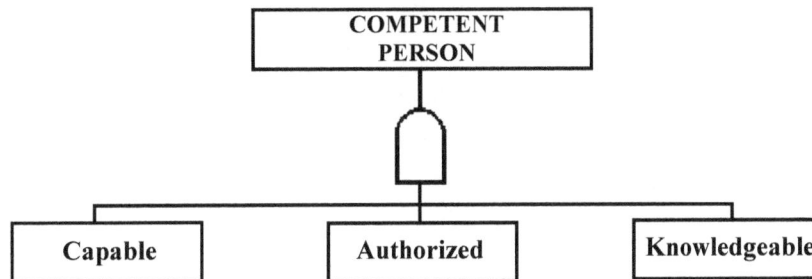

The result is a system fed by an "and" gate. The competent person must be capable "and" authorized "and" knowledgeable. Failure of any one of the elements results in a failure of the entire system.

The use of a competent person is used often in many different OSHA construction standards including; lead, rigging, welding, fall protection, training, cranes and derricks, personnel hoisting, excavations, lift-slabs, steel erection, underground construction, compressed air, demolition, ladders, asbestos, cadmium etc. However, the definition is the same in all instances.

2). Answer A:

The controlling employer, in this case the general contractor, will normally be cited if the label or MSDS is not available. However, if the MSDS is not available because the subcontractor failed to provide it, then the subcontractor shall instead be cited.

3). Answer D:

The current opinion is that the sub-contractors should develop their own procedures with help from the general contractor. This method will assure maximum standardization and flexibility while assuring effective accident prevention programs. This interface not only is effective it helps each party to understand the concerns of each other and allows both sides to develop better programs. Blind adherence to the general contractors program usually does not work and just causes problems. For example, the requirement of a general to use a particular type of fall protection or hardhat or eye protection may cause hardship for the sub-contractor. On the other hand the use of a standardized general class of fall protection, or head protection etc. is going to be required by the general, so some collaboration will be required. That is, the sub probably cannot follow your procedures to the letter, so you both might as well establish some rules everyone can live with.

4). Answer A:

The insurance industry uses EMR for workers' compensation insurance as a means of determining equitable premiums. These rating systems consider the average incident losses for a given firm's type of work and amount of payroll and predict the dollar amount of expected losses due to work-related injuries and illnesses. All 50 states, DC, Guam and Puerto Rico have worker's compensation laws. If you have an experience modifier greater than 1, you have above average losses and a less than standard performance. The EMR is based on the last 3 years loss history, not including the previous year.

5). Answer C:

Safety and the responsibility for achieving it rests with management, primarily with the organization's chief executive officer, but in a shared manner with all other managers. There has always been disagreement in management circles about just how to accomplish safety, but there has always been agreement that management of safety, like all other functions has to start at the top, and be supported by subordinate executives and managers. Supervisors, foremen and workers develop their attitude about the importance of safety & health from both formal and informal clues. A divided position by management sends a clue that management is really not all that interested in safety and its just another one of those things they have to say. Management of the safety and health effort is both an art and a science and the Director of Safety & Health is merely the steward of the function. When safety is effective the entire management team deserves the credit, likewise when it fails the entire team deserves the blame. However, the first-line supervisors are the one's primarily responsible for implementing and enforcing the company's loss control and safety and health programs.

6).   Answer D:

According to leading authorities, most materials handling accidents can be prevented by the establishment of several standard program elements. Included among these elements is training on the hazards of improper movement of materials, lifting techniques and proper conditioning. The establishment of physical requirements for strenuous materials handling applications has proven to be a valuable mishap reduction technique. Likewise, proper job placement is important in any area but certainly in the area of materials handling. Job descriptions by themselves will not produce any appreciable effect on mishaps, however the establishment of job descriptions to identify high profile jobs can be used effectively for establishing training programs, establishing physical requirements and eventually for job placement. However, this question asked about single elements in an overall effort, and selection job descriptions by themselves is the least effective element.

7).   Answer C:

1910.146(f) Entry permit: The entry permit that documents compliance with this section and authorizes entry to a permit space shall identify:
- The permit space to be entered;
- The purpose of the entry;
- The date and the authorized duration of the entry permit;
- The authorized entrants within the permit space, by name or by such other means (for example, through the use of rosters or tracking systems) as will enable the attendant to determine quickly and accurately, for the duration of the permit, which authorized entrants are inside the permit space;

8).   Answer A:

The cause factors discovered during accident investigations are normally corrected by the level of supervision that exercises control over the operation.

9). Answer C:

Accident investigation has as its primary purpose the prevention of similar occurrences and the discovery of hazards. The intent is not to place blame or administer discipline, but rather to determine how responsibilities may be defined or clarified and to reduce error producing situations. Accident investigation should improve the safety of operations, if accident investigation is used for punitive measures, the tool has the reverse effect.

10). Answer B:

The well-known principle of "span of control" is defined as that a manager cannot effectively supervise more than half a dozen subordinate managers.

11). Answer B:

OSHA requires employers to certify that they have evaluated compliance with process safety requirements at least every three years. Prompt response to audit findings and documentation that deficiencies are corrected is required. Employers must retain the two most recent audit reports. Additionally, 1910.119 requires each employer to have written operating procedures, to perform a process hazard analysis and to conduct training.

12). Answer A:

Positive reinforcement is the best motivator. Recognizing workers for reporting hazards and correcting them is a positive individual metric for safety performance.

13). Answer A:

1910.1200(b)(6) This section does not apply to: Any hazardous waste as such term is defined by the Solid Waste Disposal Act, as amended by the Resource Conservation and Recovery Act of 1976, as amended (42 U.S.C. 6901 et seq.), when subject to regulations issued under that Act by the EPA.

14). Answer B:

The best place to interview a witness during an accident investigation is the accident site, if this is not possible you want a private location that will not intimidate, inhibit or distract the witness. Your office or a supervisor's office may be intimidating.

15). Answer C:

ANSI approved the ANSI/ASSE Z10, Occupational Health & Safety Management Systems (OHSMS) consensus standard applicable to organizations of all sizes. The standard provides safety professionals and senior management with a well-conceived, state of the art concept and action outline to improve safety & health management systems. In crafting Z10, the intent was not only to achieve significant safety and health benefits through the first application, but also to impact favorably on productivity, financial performance, quality and other business goals. There is no provision specifically dedicated to regulatory compliance. The key provisions pertain to risk assessment and prioritization; applying a prescribed hierarchy of controls to achieve acceptable levels of risk levels; design reviews, management of change systems; having safety specifications in procurement systems; and safety audits.

16). Answer B:

Both Quality and EHS management systems are built on the well-known **Plan-Do-Check-Act** process. Briefly stated, the purpose of the standards is to provide organizations with an effective tool for continuous improvement in their occupational health and safety management systems to reduce the risk of occupational injuries, illnesses and fatalities.

17). Answer B:

There is no doubt that an investigator's first tasking is to get to the scene safely. Everyone is in a hurry to get to the scene of the accident, but you cannot render assistance or perform an adequate investigation if you do not arrive safely. The job of a health and safety professional cannot start until the scene is secured, meaning that the injured are taken care of and the scene itself is made safe. If you arrive earlier than this you run the risk of becoming part of the emergency services effort which tends to make you part of the response rather than part of the investigative team. There are exceptions, such as in the care of the safety engineer who is part of the rescue or re-entry team, but in most cases the advice is solid.

18).   Answer D:

A Pareto chart is used to graphically summarize and display the relative importance of the differences between groups of data. The left-side vertical axis of the pareto chart is labelled Frequency (the number of counts for each category), the right-side vertical axis of the pareto chart is the cumulative percentage, and the horizontal axis of the pareto chart is labelled with the group names of your response variables. Then determine the number of data points that reside within each group and construct the pareto chart, but unlike the bar chart, the pareto chart is ordered in descending frequency magnitude. The groups are defined by the user. The Pareto Chart Answers the following questions:

- What are the largest issues facing our team or business?
- What 20% of sources are causing 80% of the problems (80/20 Rule)?
- Where should we focus our efforts to achieve the greatest improvements?

19).   Answer B:

The term *incident* encompasses first-aid cases, recordable cases, restricted workday cases, lost-workday cases, permanent disability cases, near-misses and property damage cases. One must understand the two basic categories of cost: Direct incident costs represent actual cash outlays attributable to the incident; such outlays would not have been necessary had the incident not occurred. Examples of Direct *Costs include:* Workers' Compensation; Medical-Related Treatment; Medical Treatment Supplies; Ambulance Service; Drug Testing; Job Accommodations; and New Equipment. Indirect incident costs represent costs in terms of time and resources (other than cash) incurred as a result of the incident. Examples of Indirect *Costs include:* Healthcare Professional; Injured Worker; Supervisor; Return to Work; Incident Review; Lost Production/Productivity; Human Resources; Cost to Hire; Manager; Process Delays/Interruptions; Security; Training; and Legal. Thus, total incident costs are the sum of these costs.

20). Answer B:

1926.652(e)(1)(v): Removal shall begin at, and progress from, the bottom of the excavation. Members shall be released slowly so as to note any indication of possible failure of the remaining members of the structure or possible cave-in of the sides of the excavation.

21). Answer C:

A *supported* scaffold is considered to be inherently unstable when its height exceeds four times its width. At that height, the scaffold must be tied to the structure with guys, ties or braces. These must be installed in accordance with manufacturers' recommendations. For scaffolds more than three (3) feet wide, additional tie-ins are required every 26 vertical feet above that, but no more than 20 feet from the top of a structure; and, also every 30 feet horizontally. For scaffolds three (3) or less in width, these tie-ins are required at every 20 vertical feet.

22). Answer B:

Wood ladders shall not be coated with any opaque covering, except for identification or warning labels which may be placed on one face only of a side rail. The minimum perpendicular clearance between fixed ladder rungs, cleats, and steps, and any obstruction behind the ladder shall be 7 inches (18 cm), except in the case of an elevator pit ladder for which a minimum perpendicular clearance of 4 1/2 inches (11 cm) is required.

23). Answer B:

A tie off point is where the lanyard is attached to a structural support. This support must have 5000 lbs capacity for each worker tying off. Workers should always tie off at or above the D-ring point of the belt or harness. This ensures that the free fall is minimized, and that the lanyard doesn't interfere with personal movement. Workers must also tie off in a manner that ensures no lower level will be struck during a fall. To do this, add the height of the worker, the lanyard length, and the elongation factor of 3.5 feet. Using this formula, a six-foot tall worker requires a tie-off point at least 15.5 feet above the next lower level.

24). Answer D:

Chain inspections should be done visually in an attempt to detect any elongation or other defect. This is best accomplished by a link-by-link inspection. Overall measurements or caliper readings of a section are often misleading because not all links will be affected or damaged.

25). Answer D:

According to OSHA at 1926.250(b)(6) "Brick stacks shall not be more than 7 feet in height. When a loose brick stack reaches a height of 4 feet, it shall be tapered back 2 inches in every foot of height above the 4-foot level".

Domain 3: Quiz 3 Questions

1). While interviewing witnesses to an accident or participants in the event, investigators often find themselves talking to a hostile and very defensive people. Which of the following methods would most likely result in an honest and truthful statement from these interviewees?

    A) Inform these people that all that they say will be written down and filed; thus, telling the truth is imperative

    B) Tell them the information will only be used for accident prevention purposes and no disciplinary actions will result from the investigation

    C) Inform the person that it would be appreciated if they would tell the truth since it may help secure investigator's current position within the company and should not affect them

    D) Tell them that they are supposed to be informed of their rights, but will not be, so they have nothing to fear because anything they say cannot be used against them

2). When a new hazardous chemical has been introduced to the workplace by a subcontractor, who is expected to inform the general contractor and subcontractor workers?

    A) Superintendent

    B) Subcontractor

    C) Foreman

    D) Safety Officer

3). A modern management approach to the success of a long-term safety management system is known as?

    A) Autonomous Management

    B) Silos

    C) Team-based

    D) Empowered employees

4). A worker arrives at work with his own sunglasses stating they are "safe enough.", Supervisor should look for:

    A) Markings for ANSI Z87 on frame

    B) Proper light refraction in lenses by holding to light

    C) Nothing. Allow worker to wear sunglasses

    D) Nothing. Have worker check with Site Manager

5). You are transiting the construction site and spot a safety hazard that presents imminent danger to the workers in the area. Your first action should be to:
   A) Shut down the job site
   B) Fix the hazard
   C) Post a lock-out/tag-out sign until the hazard is corrected
   D) Notify the area supervisor to get the hazard corrected

6). In order to provide a safe work place, the safety professional should:
   A) Always seek an outside opinion before making a decision
   B) Consult the local ASSE chapter for guidance when needed
   C) Make decisions on all situations based on their knowledge
   D) Limit their advice and recommendation to those areas that they have knowledge in

7). As a new safety manager you have been ask to develop an incident data collection system, what is the most important first step in this process?
   A) Identify existing data sources and codify the data
   B) Establish incident reporting procedures.
   C) Define the subsequent use of the data.
   D) Define investigation team parameters.

8). Because of high eye and foot injury rates, management at a union labor manufacturing plant must take action. Which action should a safety professional perform first?
   A) Survey the facilities and operations to determine probable causes of the injuries.
   B) Initiate a personal protective equipment program that will include provision of both safety glasses with side shields and hard-toed shoes.
   C) Schedule a meeting with the head of the local union to review the injury problems.
   D) Charter a facility-wide safety committee.

9). In conducting a safety and health audit you ask for workers' compensation cost data and find the location's experience modification rate to be 0.55. How would you rate the location's safety and health performance with respect to this measure?

    A) Excellent
    B) Good
    C) Fair
    D) Poor

10). An CHST goes into an area with several unsafe conditions involving different contractors. The CHST should:

    A) Allow work to continue
    B) Write a report to the project manager
    C) Submit a report to OSHA
    D) Stop work and discuss with the contractors supervisors

11). The work crew notices contractor employees in an area they are not normally working in and notifies the supervisor. The supervisor should:

    A) Report to Site Manager
    B) Stop work and ask contractor employees what they are doing
    C) Continue work and observe contractor employees for safety violations
    D) Assume they are supposed to be there and continue work

12). During an inspection of your site an OSHA Compliance Officer refuses to wear a hard hat in one area because he says there is no overhead hazard. However, your company rules require the wearing of hardhats throughout the complex and this area is no exception. Does the OSHA Compliance Officer have the right to refuse to wear the PPE?

    A) No, but since the rule is stupid, forget it
    B) Yes, he is OSHA and can do whatever he wants
    C) No, the OSHA Compliance Officer must abide by your rules
    D) Yes, if OSHA does not require a hardhat you cannot force a federal employee to abide by your rules

13). During an OSHA inspection of your site, who determines what areas will be visited and for how long?
   A) The OSHA Compliance Officer
   B) The employee representative
   C) A Certified Health & Safety Technician
   D) The owner

14). An employer cited by OSHA has a period of _____ to contest the citation. The notice to contest is sent directly to the _____.
   A) 15 working days, OSHA Area Director
   B) 10 working days, Occupation Safety & Health Review Commission
   C) 15 working days, Occupation Safety & Health Review Commission
   D) 15 working days, OSHA Regional Administrator

15). Under what conditions should a safety professional exert functional authority?
   A) never
   B) always
   C) during startup operations
   D) when line management fails to provide adequate leadership

16). The best selection of people for a safety committee is:
   A) Upper and mid-level manager
   B) Supervisors and line workers
   C) Company owners and shareholders
   D) Contractors and government officials

17). A staff safety engineer is given the authority by the General Manager to stop operations on a construction site whenever he or she observes an imminent danger situation. Which of the following correctly identifies the authority granted by the General Manager?
   A) Staff authority
   B) Staff to line authority
   C) Authority of delegation
   D) Functional authority

18). If an OSHA Compliance Safety & Health Officer (CSHO) is inspecting your site and you refuse to allow him/her to inspect a particular area, what is the CSHO supposed to do?
   A) Stop the inspection immediately and obtain a federal warrant served by a federal marshal
   B) Continue the inspection, you have the right to limit the inspection to any area of the site you wish
   C) Continue the inspection and report the refusal to the area director
   D) Stop the inspection and issue you a citation for obstruction of a federal officer

19). In determining if a serious violation exists, the CSHO finds that the supervisor had full knowledge of the hazard. Does this knowledge constitute a serious violation?
   A) No, the supervisor is considered an employee not the employer
   B) Yes, the supervisor represents the employer and a supervisor's knowledge of the hazard amounts to employer knowledge
   C) No, the supervisor could have chosen not have told the owner
   D) Yes, the owner should have known if he would have been doing his job

20). An OSHA Compliance officer arrives at your facility to conduct an inspection. Which of the following is the CSHO not required to provide?
   A) their official identification
   B) scope of the inspection
   C) identify the records to be reviewed
   D) the name of the individual that issued the complaint

21). A project is requiring long work hours for multiple weeks to meet a production deadline. You observe an equipment operator falling asleep between lifts, the **best** course of action is to:
   A) Enter the operator on safety report.
   B) Instruct the rigger to ensure to wake the operator
   C) Recommend to management to review work rest cycle
   D) Send an email or text reminding the operator of the importance of safety

22). Safety professionals sometimes incorrectly use the terms risk and hazard interchangeably. Risk is **best** defined as:
    A) Conditions of things.
    B) Actions or inactions of people.
    C) A measure of the probability and severity of adverse effects.
    D) Any workplace condition that can result in injury, death, or property damage.

23). Who is most responsible for ensuring a union worker follows safety rules?
    A) Union Steward
    B) OSHA
    C) Union representative on safety committee
    D) Employer

24). You are working for the general contractor and assisting sub-contractors with job safety analysis on a multiemployer jobsite. The Electricians identified a new Pipefitter task that would assists the Plumbers with installing water lines. The Pipefitters stated that the union agreement precluded them from assisting the Plumbers. What is the best course of action to resolve the issue of task responsibility?
    A) Assign the responsibility to all trades
    B) Negotiate the tasks with the union representatives.
    C) Assign the task responsibility to only the Pipefitters.
    D) Notify the general site management staff to resolve the issue and communicate the policy to the appropriate parties.

25). How can line management help ensure line supervisors are held accountable for safety performance?
    A) Develop a culture where management relies on self-directed work teams to enforce safety accountability among work groups.
    B) Build written management safety policies and enforcement principles into line supervisor accountability.
    C) Require management safety policies to prescribe line supervisors as the point-of-contact for line safety.
    D) Perform training for all employees identifying line supervisors as the principle enforcement agent for line safety.

Domain 3: Quiz 3 Answers

1) Answer B:

Dealing with hostile, belligerent or dishonest witnesses or participants, is a way of life for accident investigators. There are many theories about obtaining frank, candid and honest statements from these people. However, it is generally accepted that the most effective way is to explain that your investigation is for accident prevention purposes only and cannot be used for any type of disciplinary action. This tends to set the person at ease and will usually result in more open and honest responses about the mishap. However, investigators must be sure that they are telling the truth about purposes of the report. Often statements made in safety investigations wind up in personnel files or personnel action documents. Thus, assurance that investigative reports are only used for accident prevention purposes is essential. Do not provide false guarantees regarding use of the information. Develop a policy concerning safety investigation prior to the need!

2) Answer B:

Any employer that introduces a new hazardous chemical into the multi-employer workplace must inform the general contractor and affected sub-contractor workers.

3) Answer C:

A Team-based approach to safety management is a modern management model used to continuously improve a safety management system.

4) Answer A:

ANSI approves specifications for safety glasses. The markings for ANSI Z87 on frames are the indicator that they meet ANSI standards for impact lenses.

5) Answer D:

The person to correct the hazard should be the individual with the most knowledge of the area, that is the area supervisor.

6)   Answer D:

This can be a difficult question, but the BEST answer of those listed it to only make recommendations if you are sure that the result will ensure a safer work area. Making recommendations about areas that you are not skill in has the potential to be incorrect.

7).   Answer C:

In the book *Safety Culture and Effective Safety Management,* author Swartz explains that before collecting data and developing a system to collect and manipulate the data, it is essential to define how the data will be used.

8).   Answer A:

In *Accident Prevention Manual for Business and Industry: Administration and Programs,* A key part of risk management is investigating incidents and taking corrective actions based upon the facts associated with the incidents. An essential aspect of the investigation process is understanding the causal factors and the subsequent root causes that had to the incidents so appropriate corrective actions can be identified and implemented.

9).   Answer A:

The experience modification is developed from the location's injury/illness frequency and severity rate and the industry rate. If the plant had the same experience as the industry as a whole the experience modification rate would be 1. Since this plant had an experience modification rate of 0.55 it would be considered excellent.

10).   Answer D:

The best approach is to stop the work and discuss the situation with supervisors from all contractors involved with the operation in question.

11). Answer B:

A supervisor should suspend operations and investigate suspicious activity from other contracting crews.

12). Answer C:

29 CFR 1903.7(c) requires that the OSHA Compliance Officer comply with all safety and health rules and practices at the establishment and wear or use the safety clothing or protective equipment required by OSHA standards or by the employer for the protection of employees.

13). Answer A:

The employer has the right to refuse entry to an OSHA Compliance Officer or to limit the scope of that inspection as a refusal of entry. However assuming that the employer does not choose to restrict the OSHA Compliance Officer, the route, timing and scope of inspection is largely up to the inspector. Inspections are either comprehensive or partial. Comprehensive inspections would of course include virtually everything a wall-to-wall inspection. Partial inspections are limited to certain potentially hazardous areas, operations, conditions or practices at the site. These partial inspections can be expanded based on information gathered by the OSHA Compliance Officer during the inspection process.

14). Answer A:

When OSHA provides a penalty for a citation, they do it by certified mail. From the time you receive the letter you have 15 working days to contest the citation or the proposed assessment of penalty or both. You must notify the OSHA Area Director within this 15-day period or both the citation and penalty become final. The OSHA Area Director then forwards your notice to the Occupational Safety and Health Review Commission.

15). Answer D:

The granting of temporary functional authority is common and necessary. The safety staff works best by influencing the line, not directing it. However, if line management is failing to do it job in a safe manner, then it is proper to give the safety staff function authority.

16). Answer B:

A Safety committee should be a good representation of the organization. Supervisors and workers are critical members of a safety committee.

17). Answer D:

The operational control delegated the safety engineer to shut down dangerous jobs by the General Manager is functional or line authority. This authority, or lack of it, is hotly debated by safety and health professionals. One position calls the delegation of such power unnecessary. This opinion states that even the threat of a shutdown is most certainly going to be a confrontational issue. An issue that will eventually have to be resolved by higher authority and that often leads to long lasting negative relations between staff and operations. The other side of this debate feels they need the reserve strength over line managers because of the conflict between organizational demands and safety concerns. They further advance the argument by noting that the act of delegation of authority is in itself a strong commitment by senior management to the safety process.

18). Answer C:

OSHA provides the following instruction to the OSHA Compliance Safety & Health Officers in the Field Inspection Reference Manual. "If the employer refuses to allow an inspection of the establishment to proceed, the CSHO shall leave the premises and immediately report the refusal to the Assistant Area Director. The Area Director shall notify the Regional Solicitor. If the employer raises no objection to inspection of certain portions of the workplace but objects to inspection of other portions, this shall be documented. Normally, the CSHO shall continue the inspection, confining it only to those certain portions to which the employer has raised no objections. In either case the CSHO shall advise the employer that the refusal will be reported to the Assistant Area Director and that the agency may take further action, which may include obtaining legal process."

19). Answer B:

Section 17(k) of the OSHAct explains that: " a serious violation shall be deemed to exist in a place of employment if there is a substantial probability that death or serious physical harm could result from a condition which exists, or from one or more practices, means, methods, operations, or processes which have been adopted or are in use, in such place of employment unless the employer did not, and could not with the exercise of reasonable diligence, know of the presence of the violation."

In determining if a hazard is serious or not the question was "**Whether the employer knew**, or with the exercise of reasonable diligence, could have known of the presence of the hazardous condition." In this regard, the supervisor represents the employer and a supervisor's knowledge of the hazardous condition amounts to employer knowledge. In cases where the employer may contend that the supervisor's own conduct constitutes an isolated event of employee misconduct, the CSHO will attempt to determine the extent to which the supervisor was trained and supervised so as to prevent such conduct, and how the employer enforces the rule. If, after reasonable attempts to do so, it cannot be determined that the employer has actual knowledge of the hazardous condition, the knowledge requirement is met in the eyes of OSHA if the CSHO is satisfied that the employer could have known through the exercise of reasonable diligence. As a general rule, if the CSHO was able to discover a hazardous condition, and the condition was not transitory in nature, it can be presumed that the employer could have discovered the same condition through the exercise of reasonable diligence.

20). Answer D:

The compliance officer must provide official identification upon arrival.
At the opening conference, the CSHO will:
- inform the employer the purpose of the visit.
- provide the employer copies of the Act, standards or regulations, as required.

Outline in general terms:

- scope of the inspection
- records the officer wants to review
- the officer's obligation to confer with employees
- physical inspection of the workplace

- closing conference
- if applicable, furnish the employer with a copy of any complaint, if it is the reason for the inspection (the name of the individual or individuals will not be revealed).
- answer questions

21). Answer C:

The professional role of a risk/safety manager is to implement and evaluate the effectiveness of risk management program and report finding and recommendations to decision makers and key shareholders. Communication is a vital management component to any organization. Whether the purpose is to update employees on new policies, to prepare for a weather disaster, to ensure safety throughout the organization or to listen to the attitudes of employees, effective communication is an integral issue in effective management.

22) Answer C:

A hazard is defined as a condition, set of circumstances, or inherent property that can cause injury, illness, or death. Risk is an estimation of the combination of the likelihood of an occurrence of a hazardous event or exposure(s), and the severity of injury or illness that may be caused by the event or exposures. Risk assessment is a process(s) used to evaluate the level of risk associated with hazards and system issues. A risk assessment matrix provides a qualitative method to categorize combinations of indicators for occurrence probability and severity outcome, thus establishing risk levels. A matrix provides an effective visual tool and helps in communication with decision makers when deciding on the actions to be taken to reduce the risk. Risk assessment matrices can also be used to compare and prioritize risks, and to effectively allocate mitigation resources. (ANSI/ASSE Z10-2012)

23) Answer D:

Line supervisor is the most able and responsible for ensuring workers follow safety rules. Ultimately, it is the employer's responsibility to determine appropriate policy and procedures and enforce the rules.

24) Answer D:

It is important for a safety professional to realize when issues are beyond his/her control. For management/labor operational conflicts, it is best to direct the issue to management for resolution.

25) Answer B:

In Peterson's *Techniques of Safety Management: A Systems Approach,* 4th Edition, Line supervisors will do what they perceive is being measured and what they perceived they will be rewarded for doing. Therefore, written expectations and written policies for enforcement and accountability should be incorporated into line supervision at every level of management.

Domain 3: Quiz 4 Questions

1). As a CHST, you are expected to
   A) Ensure the profitability of company as your priority.
   B) Seek methods to improve personal knowledge and understanding of methods, techniques and practices for workers' protection.
   C) Seek to improve personal knowledge of financial and accounting practices related to supervising construction activities.
   D) Carefully assess situation and problems to identify the most productive methods of completing construction tasks, while working to maintain work area in a manner that will pass regulatory inspection.

2). Which action is preferred when dealing with minor infractions of work safety rules?
   A) Oral reprimand
   B) Written reprimand
   C) No response or consequence
   D) Suspension

3). What should a supervisor do when a crew must walk across as area with open floor holes to get to their work area?
   A) Warn them of hazards and tell them to avoid the holes.
   B) Let them walk through.
   C) Have floor holes covered before allowing workers to walk across.
   D) Have the floor holes covered and inform crew of load surface restrictions.

4). Both large and small businesses are required to report certain serious work-related incidents to nearest OSHA Area Office. What mishaps require reporting within 8 hours?
   A) The first aid injury of an employee that required hospitalization, as a result of a work-related incident
   B) The fatality of one or more employees, as a result of a work-related incident
   C) The injury of more than three employees that requires hospitalization or involves traumatic amputation or broken bones, as a result of a work-related incident
   D) The transport of five or more workers to a hospital, as a result of a work-related incident

5). Often several accident investigators will be at the scene of an accident at the same time due varying reasons for gathering information. Which of the following is the **least** important task with respect to the CHSTs accident investigation responsibilities?

    A) Getting to the scene before anybody else Arriving first on the scene

    B) Preventing a second accident

    C) Preserving as much evidence as possible

    D) Taking care of, and/or transporting the injured and/or dead

6). A contractor has proposed several options for developing and complying with safety and health procedures while reviewing a bid for a large construction job. Which of the following will produce the most effective safety and health interface?

    A) The sub-contractor should develop their own procedures and follow them to the letter

    B) The sub-contractor should use the general contractor's procedures to provide site standardization

    C) The sub-contractor should follow all OSHA rules and, thus, will not need procedures

    D) The sub-contractor should develop their own procedures with assistance from general contractor

7). A CHST observes the back of a rough terrain fork truck lift off the ground as a heavy load is being lifted on a job site. Which of the following is the **FIRST** course of action?

    A) Direct the crew to add extra counter weight to stabilize the operation.

    B) Stop the crew and advise to discontinue with the lift.

    C) Instruct the crew to add air to load side tires.

    D) Direct the operator to tip mast back once load is lifted.

8). When transiting the production area, a supervisor spots a safety hazard in a different department that presents imminent danger to contracted workers in the area. His/her first action should be to:

    A) Shut down production line and file a report

    B) Bring the issue up in the next meeting.

    C) Post a lock-out/tag-out sign until hazard is corrected

    D) Stop the work and notify area supervisor to get hazard corrected

9). During an accident investigation, which of the following is an indirect cost?

    A) Workers compensation cost.

    B) Loss productivity.

    C) Medical costs.

    D) Repairing property damage.

10). An operation requiring scaffolding presents overhead fall hazards above workers. Workers of different contractors are assigned to various levels in the scaffold. The responsibility for protecting workers from the overhead hazards belongs to:

    A) All workers on scaffold.

    B) Workers on top of scaffold.

    C) Workers below top level of scaffold.

    D) Contracting employers.

11). On a multi-employer steel erection project, the entity that has the overall responsibility for the construction of the project-its planning, quality, and completion is the:

    A) Qualified person.

    B) Project superintendent.

    C) Controlling contractor.

    D) Competent person.

12). The crew must perform work along a train track. What should be the best approach to doing the work safely?

    A) Try to use an old Job Safety Analysis (JSA) used by railroad.

    B) Use your JSA and incorporating railroad hazards from it.

    C) Just go to work.

    D) Coordinate with railroad, review JSA prior to performing work, and post train schedules at jobsite.

13). At what exposure level are you required to wear hearing protection for an 8-hour exposure?
   A) 85 dBA
   B) 90 dBA
   C) 80 dBA
   D) Using hearing protection in construction increases the chances of being injured because you cannot hear what is going on around you

14). A Waiver of Subrogation clause is?
   A) Waiving Maranda rights
   B) Waiving the right to sue your employer
   C) Waiving the right to pass on liability to a subcontractor
   D) Waiving a hold harmless agreement

15). Individual susceptibility to heat-related illness can vary widely between workers. New workers and those returning from a prolonged absence should be expected to do how much of the work load after 4 days?
   A) 20%
   B) 50%
   C) 60%
   D) 100%

16). When an injured worker returns to work after a prolonged period of being away, they may combat acute dehydration, illness, or fatigue. Supervisors should to make adjustments to the worker's workload for how many days so the worker has time to re-acclimatize?
   A) 1 day
   B) 2 days
   C) 3 days
   D) 4 days

17). What is the best risk assessment method for tower crane erection?
   A) FMEA
   B) Fault tree
   C) HAZOP
   D) JSA

18). Who responsible if worker chooses to use his own gear?
   A) The employee to verify it is right for the hazards on the job
   B) OHSA to verify it is right for the hazards on the job
   C) Employer/supervisor to verify it is right for the hazards on the job
   D) Employees are never allowed to use their own gear

19). What is the best benchmark for comparing companies' performance to the industry?
   A) Drug testing positive rate
   B) Employee injury rate
   C) Equipment damage rate
   D) EMR

20). Which two concepts are involved with "chain of custody"?
   A) Possession / control
   B) Ownership / accountability
   C) Blame / evidence
   D) Tampering / gathering

21). What is the most appropriate question to ask at the end of an accident investigation interview?
   A) Why do you think he did it?
   B) Who do you think could have prevented this?
   C) What do you think are the root causes?
   D) Why do you think this happened?

22). Most often, the Root Cause of an incident is:
   A) Management system failure
   B) Employee negligence
   C) Lack of commitment by safety people
   D) Lack of rules & regulations

23). Based on the illustrated Hazard Grid, what would be your assigned **priority** of hazards?

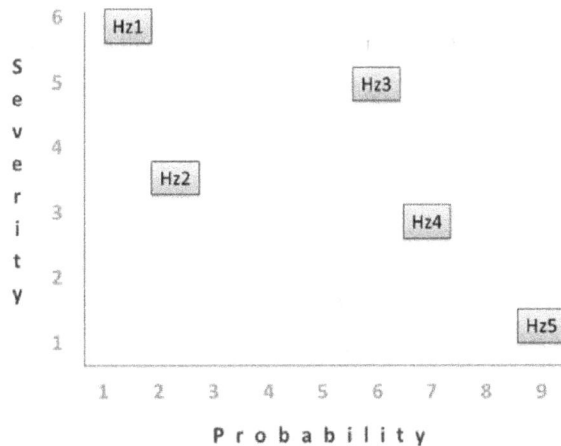

A) Hz1, Hz2, Hz3, Hz4, Hz5.
B) Hz1, Hz3, Hz2, Hz4, Hz5.
C) Hz5, Hz4, Hz3, Hz2, Hz1.
D) Hz3, Hz4, Hz1, Hz5, Hz2.

24). What is the ratio between direct costs and indirect cost?
A) 1:4
B) 1:5
C) 3:1
D) 2:1

25). The "5 whys" of incident investigation method is most closely related to which type of analysis?
A) Cause and effect.
B) JSA.
C) FMEA.
D) Root cause.

Domain 3: Quiz 4 Answers

1)   Answer B:

Seek methods to improve your knowledge and understanding of methods, techniques and practices for protection of workers. STS Code of Ethics

2)   Answer A:

Progressive companies believe the proper way to deal with minor rule infractions is to issue an oral reprimand for the first offense. Progressive discipline is then administered for additional violations.

3)   Answer D:

Have the floor holes covered and inform your crew of the load surface restrictions.

4)   Answer B:

Employers have to report the following events to OSHA:
- All work-related fatalities
- All work-related in-patient hospitalizations of one or more employees
- All work-related amputations
- All work-related losses of an eye

Employers must report work-related fatalities within **8 hours of finding out about it.**

For any in-patient hospitalization, amputation, or eye loss employers must report the incident within 24 hours of learning about it.

Only fatalities occurring within 30 days of the work-related incident must be reported to OSHA. Further, for an inpatient hospitalization, amputation or loss of an eye, then incidents must be reported to OSHA only if they occur within 24 hours of the work-related incident.

Each report required by this section shall relate the following information:
- Establishment name
- location of incident
- Time of incident
- Number of fatalities or hospitalized employee(s)
- Name(s) of injured employee(s)
- Contact person

- Phone number
- Description of incident

5)   Answer A:

There is no doubt that an investigator's first task is to arrive at the scene safely. All responders are in a hurry to get to the scene of the accident, but cannot render assistance or perform an adequate investigation if they do not arrive safely. The job of a health and safety professional cannot start until the scene is secured, meaning that the injured are taken care of and the scene itself is made safe. If responders arrive prior to scene security, they run the risk of becoming part of the emergency services effort, making them part of the response, rather than part of the investigative team. There are exceptions, such as in the case of the safety engineer who is part of a rescue or re-entry team, but in most cases, safe arrival to the scene is paramount.

6)   Answer D:

The current opinion is that the sub-contractors should develop their own procedures, with help from the general contractor. This method will assure maximum standardization and flexibility, while assuring effective accident prevention programs. This interface is not only effective, but helps each party to understand each other's concerns and allows both sides to develop better programs. Blind adherence to general contractors' programs usually does not work and causes further problems. For example, the requirement of a general contractor to use a particular type of fall protection or hardhat or eye protection may cause hardship for the sub-contractor. On the other hand, the use of a standardized general class of fall protection, or head protection is going to be required by general contractors, so some collaboration will be required. That is, the sub-contractor probably cannot follow procedures to the letter, so sub-contractors and general contractors should establish basic rules that all people involved can live with.

7)   Answer B:

A fork truck should never be operated with an overload. This condition removes weight from the steering wheels, which affects control of the machine. Never add counterweight because it can seriously overload the forks, tires, axles, chains etc.

8)   Answer D:

If workers are in eminent danger, the best is to stop the work and notify the direct supervisor. The person to correct the hazard should be the individual with the most area knowledge, that is, the area supervisor.

9)   Answer B:

Loss productivity would be considered an indirect cost to the incident.

10)   Answer D:

To protect employees from falling hand tools, debris, and other small objects, install toeboards, screens, guardrail systems, debris nets, catch platforms, canopy structures, or barricades. In addition, employees must wear hard hats. 1926.451(h)(1) & (2) and (3). With multiple contractors on the scaffold, each employer has responsibilities for protecting their workers from overhead fall hazards.

11)   Answer C:

In the OSHA Steel Erection Standard, the controlling contractor has specific responsibilities. Controlling contractor means a prime contractor, general contractor, construction manager or any other legal entity that has the overall responsibility for the construction of the project-it's planning, quality, and completion. (2016). OSHA Steel Erection Controlling Contractor Requirements. *OSHA Steel Erection eTool*. Retrieved 3/15/2016, OSHA Steel Erection eTool

The standard placed these duties on the controlling contractor because, as the contractor with general supervisory authority over the worksite, it is in the best position to comply with them. None of these provisions require the controlling contractor to direct the individual employees of a subcontractor or supplier. The extent of the measures that a controlling employer must implement to satisfy this duty of reasonable care is less than what is required of an employer with respect to protecting its own employees. This means that the controlling employer is not normally required to inspect for hazards as frequently or to have the same level of knowledge of the applicable standards or of trade expertise as the employer it has hired.

(2016). OSHA Letter of Interpretation Controlling Contractors. Retrieved 5/15/2016, OSHA

12)   Answer D:

Coordinate with the railroad, review JSA prior to performing work, and post train schedules at jobsite.

13)   Answer A:

85 decibels (A-weighted) or dBA 85 is the "Action Level" where hearing protection is required.

14)   Answer C:

The term "subrogate" means to take legal action against someone else. Typically it is used in cases where one party is taking action against a third party, such as a car insurance agency recovering funds from another agency or third person because the agency has paid to repair their client's car that was damaged by the third person or other agency. A waiver of subrogation is verbiage in a contract that prevents legal liability being passed to the third party.

15)   Answer D:

CDC/NIOSH Science Blog: "Upon return, the worker may combat acute dehydration, illness, or fatigue so supervisors need to make adjustments so the worker has time to re-acclimatize. This can take 2 to 3 days when returning to a hot job." https://blogs.cdc.gov/niosh-science-blog/2014/07/14/acclimatization/

OSHA: "Develop a heat acclimatization program and plans that promote work at a steady moderate rate that can be sustained in the heat. For example, new workers and those returning from a prolonged absence should begin with 20% of the workload on the first day, increasing incrementally by no more than 20% each subsequent day. During a rapid change leading to excessively hot weather or conditions such as a heat wave, even experienced workers should begin on the first day of work in excessive heat with 50% of the normal workload and time spent in the hot environment, 60% on the second day, 80% on day three, and 100% on the fourth day. Full acclimatization may take up to 14 days or longer depending on factors relating to the individual, such as increased risk of heat illness due to certain medications or medical conditions, or the environment." *https://www.osha.gov/SLTC/heatillness/heat_index/acclimatizing_workers.html*

16)   Answer D:

CDC/NIOSH Science Blog: "Upon return, the worker may combat acute dehydration, illness, or fatigue so supervisors need to make adjustments so the worker has time to re-acclimatize. This can take 2 to 3 days when returning to a hot job." https://blogs.cdc.gov/niosh-science-blog/2014/07/14/acclimatization/

OSHA: "Develop a heat acclimatization program and plans that promote work at a steady moderate rate that can be sustained in the heat. For example, new workers and those returning from a prolonged absence should begin with 20% of the workload on the first day, increasing incrementally by no more than 20% each subsequent day. During a rapid change leading to excessively hot weather or conditions such as a heat wave, even experienced workers should begin on the first day of work in excessive heat with 50% of the normal workload and time spent in the hot environment, 60% on the second day, 80% on day three, and 100% on the fourth day. Full acclimatization may take up to 14 days or longer depending on factors relating to the individual, such as increased risk of heat illness due to certain medications or medical conditions, or the environment." *https://www.osha.gov/SLTC/heatillness/heat_index/acclimatizing_workers.html*

17)   Answer A:

Failure modes and effects analysis (FMEA): System analysis technique that identifies the manner in which failures occur and investigates their impact on one another, as well as on other parts of the system. FMEA is usually applied to a complex mechanical situation or electrical equipment.

Fault-tree analysis (FTA): System safety technique using deductive (general to specific) analysis that starts with an undesired event and analyzes the way the undesired event can occur. Uses Boolean algebra to simplify the fault-tree diagram to a minimal cut set, which is the shortest, most direct path that allows an event to take place.

Hazard and operability study (HAZOP): Study used to identify problems associated with potential hazards and deviations in plant operations from the design specifications and is carried out by a multidisciplinary team following a structure that includes a series of guide words. HAZOP is typically used with chemical management processes.

Job Safety Analysis (JSA): is a systematic analysis of job elements. It results in an in-depth evaluation by workers and first line supervisors of the individual steps and hazards. JSAs also offer protective measures or solutions to identified hazards.

18) Answer C:

It is **always** the employer's responsibility to ensure that equipment is used and maintained properly, regardless of who purchases or owns equipment on the worksite.

19) Answer B:

Injury rates are lagging indicators; however, they are perhaps the most useful metric for comparing performance between companies throughout an industry. EMR is the Experience Modification Rate which is used by the insurance industry for workers' compensation insurance as a means of determining equitable premiums.

20) Answer A:

Chain of custody (CoC) generally refers to the documentation (paper trail) of how some sort of property (generally evidence of some nature) is transported or transferred. The purpose is to track the control of the item or items so that how it was handled and who handled it is known. The main concerns are who had possession or access and who was responsible for control of the item or access to it. CoC is typically associated with evidence, but not blame. It is not about ownership or about gathering evidence, with the possible exception of documenting the pertinent data regarding when/where it was first collected. It is about accountability of preserving the sanctity of evidence and preventing tampering.

21) Answer C:

Of the options given, 'what do you think are the root causes' is the best question to ask because it forces the respondent to think about causation rather than blame and answer in discussion type answers.

22) Answer A:

Of the options given, "management system failure" is the best response. Generally, the popular philosophy in safety management is that when an adverse event occurs, management either should have known something but did not OR management knew about it but did nothing about it. Either way, there was a management system failure.

23) Answer D:

The provided 'Hazard Grid' is just one example of a risk matrix. A Risk Matrix is a formalized method of ranking potential hazards by comparing their potential (probability) against their consequences (severity). One variable (either potential or consequences) is quantified on the X axis while the other is quantified on the Y axis. The quantification (number value) is not important in itself (any numbers could be assigned) so long as they are listed in increasing order AND the same numbers are used for all hazards. Once the hazards are listed on the matrix, their associated 'risk' is calculated by their probability times their severity. That way they can all be ranked against each other and prioritized according to their anticipated impact (risk score) to the organization.

In this example, Hz1's score is 9 (1.5x6=9); Hz2 is 6.25 (2.5x2.5=6.25); Hz3 is 30 (6x5); Hz4 is 21 (3x7) and Hz5 is 9 (9x1). So, they are ranked 3-4-5-1-2. Technically, 5 and 1 have the same score but we ranked 1 ahead of 5 because while their score is the same, 1's consequences are quite a bit higher than 5's and 'ties' always go to the 'runner'—the employee. A high potential for a small cut should never out-weigh a small potential for death or disabling injury.

24) Answer A:

The indirect to direct costs ratio varies widely based on the organization, industry and even the actual incident being examined; however, a general average has been accepted to be around 4:1 (indirect to direct) since Herbert William Heinrich's published works on the topic. OSHA uses a range of ratios in their "$afety Pays" application beginning at 4.5 on the high side and 1.1 on the low side (based on total expenses).

-https://www.osha.gov/dcsp/smallbusiness/safetypays/background.html

25) Answer D:

The "5 whys" method is commonly associated with root cause analysis.

Domain 4: Leadership, Communication and Training

Management Leadership

An effective Occupational Safety and Health Management System (OHSMS) requires leadership and commitment from top management. Management leadership provides the motivating force and the resources for organizing and controlling activities within an organization. In an effective OHSMS holds worker safety and health as a fundamental value of the organization. Ideally, this means that concern for every aspect of the safety and health of all workers throughout the job site is demonstrated.

Effective leadership:

- Creates safety and health management system policy and procedures.
- Establishes and communicates organizational goals and the pathways (objectives) to achieve goals
- Demonstrates visible management involvement
- Assigns and communicating responsibility, authority and resources to responsible parties and holding those parties accountable.
- Encourages employees to report hazards, symptoms, injuries and illnesses, and identify programs or policies which discourage this reporting.

Successful top managers, superintendents, and supervisors use a variety of techniques that visibly involve them in the safety and health protection of their workers. Managers and supervisors should look for methods that fit their style and workplace conditions.

Examples of visible safety leadership:

- Getting out where you can be seen, informally or through formal inspections.
- Being accessible by incorporating safety and health into operational conversations and standard operating procedures.
- Promptly reward acceptable safety performance and correct at risk situations.
- Leading by example, by knowing and following the rules employees are expected to follow.
- Active involvement by participating in the workplace safety and health solutions.

Ten Principles of Safety Management[21]

1).	An unsafe act, an unsafe condition, and an accident are all symptoms management systems problems.
2).	Circumstances that will produce severe injuries are predictable and can be identified and controlled.
3).	Safety should be managed like any other company function. Management should direct the safety effort by setting achievable goals and by planning, organizing, and controlling to achieve them.
4).	The key to effective line safety performance is management procedures that fix accountability.

5).	The function of safety is to locate and define the operational errors that allow accidents to occur. This function can be carried out in two ways:
	  A) by asking why accidents happen - searching for their root causes
	  B) by asking whether certain known effective controls are being utilized

6).	The causes of unsafe behavior can be identified and classified. Some of the classifications are Overload (the improper matching of a person's capacity with the load); Traps, and the worker's decision to error. Each cause is one which can be controlled.
7).	In most cases, unsafe behavior is normal human behavior; it is the result of normal people reacting to their environment. Management's job is to change the environment that leads to unsafe behavior.
8).	There are three major subsystems that must be dealt with in building an effective safety system: the physical; the managerial; the behavioral
9).	The safety system should fit the culture of the organization.
10).	There is no one right way to achieve safety in an organization; however, for a safety system to be effective, the system must: Force supervisory performance; involve middle management; Have top management visibly showing their commitment; Have employee participation; be flexible; be perceived as positive.

---

[21] Adapted from Dan Peterson, 2003.

The Safety Professional

A *safety professional* is one who applies the expertise gained from a study of safety science, principles, and other subjects and from professional safety experience to create or develop procedures, processes, standards, specifications, and systems to achieve optimal control or reduction of the hazards and exposures that may harm people, property or the environment.

A *Certified Safety Professional* is a safety professional who has met and continues to meet the criteria established by the Board of Certified Safety Professionals (BCSP) and is authorized by the BCSP to use the credentials.

To perform their professional functions, individuals practicing in the safety profession generally have education, training and experience from a common body of knowledge. They need to have a fundamental knowledge of physics, chemistry, biology, physiology, statistics, mathematics, compute r science, engineering mechanics, industrial processes, business, communication and psychology.

Professional safety studies include industrial hygiene and toxicology, design of engineering hazard controls, fire protection, ergonomics, system and process safety, safety and health program management, accident investigation and analysis, product safety, construction safety, education and training methods, measurement of safety performance, human behavior, environmental safety and health, and safety, health and environmental laws, regulations and standards. Many have backgrounds or advanced study in other disciplines, such as management and business administration, engineering, education, physical and social sciences and other fields. Others have advanced study in safety, and this additional background extends their expertise beyond the basics of the safety profession.

Because safety is an element in all human endeavors, the performance of these functions, in a variety of contexts in both public and private sectors, often employ specialized knowledge and skills. Typical settings are manufacturing, insurance, risk management, government, education, consulting, construction, healthcare, engineering and design, waste management , petroleum, facilities management, retail, transportation and utilities. Within these contexts, they must adapt their functions to fit the mission, operations and climate of their employer. Not only must individuals practicing in the safety profession acquire the knowledge and skills to perform these functions effectively in their employment context, through continuing education and training they stay current with new technologies, changes in laws and regulations, and changes in the workforce, workplace and world business, political and social climate.

As part of their positions, these individuals must plan for and manage resources and funds related to their functions. They may be responsible for supervising a diverse staff of professionals. By acquiring the knowledge and skills of the profession, developing the mind set and wisdom to act responsibly in the employment context, and keeping up with changes that affect the safety profession, the required safety professional functions are able to be performed with confidence, competence and respected authority. (ANSI/ASSE Z590)

Professional Codes of Conduct

Ethics is a rational reflection upon good and evil (without weighing in on the question of heaven or hell, angels and demons). The word *ethics* refers to our identification of the "good" in any given situation as well as the rationale for the identification.

Ethics engages each of us at the level of the thought, the reasoning process that goes into every decision we make, whether for our own happiness or that of another. Sound ethical judgment arises when proper habits of thought have given way to confidence in the right conduct and in doing it.
As safety consultants (and mature adults), there is no flight from precisely this kind of deliberation. We have to make choices that are responsible, defensible, and appropriate. Decide upon the highest good and order all of the others, the lesser goods, in a hierarchy. This could be applied to a risk assessment or matrix.

There are rigorous professional guidelines and regulations regarding ethics for a safety professional. Below is a list of some of them:

- Board of Certified Safety Professionals Code of Ethics and Professional Conduct
- American Society of Safety Engineers' Code of Professional Conduct
- American Industrial Hygiene Association and American Conference of Governmental Industrial Hygienists Joint Ethical Principles
- American Board of Industrial Hygiene Code of Ethics
- International Code of Ethics for Occupational Health Professionals
- Federal Contractor Code of Business Ethics and Conduct (48 CFR 3.10)

- American Society of Civil Engineers Code of Ethics
- National Society of Professional Engineers Code of Ethics
- Institute of Hazardous Materials Management Code of Ethics

As a safety professional you should be familiar with the codes of conduct pertinent to your work. However, in and of themselves, they are insufficient. You must also develop a robust code of personal ethics. The avoidance of wrong is not the same as doing right. As safety professionals we must honor a high ethical standard, one that encompasses not just ourselves but our clients, colleagues, and community. You must not only behave ethically; you must strive to encourage ethical behavior in others.

BCSP Code of Ethics Standards:
HOLD paramount the safety and health of people, the protection of the environment and protection of property in the performance of professional duties and exercise their obligation to advise employers, clients, employees, the public, and appropriate authorities of danger and unacceptable risks to people, the environment, or property.
BE honest, fair, and impartial; act with responsibility and integrity. Adhere to high standards of ethical conduct with balanced care for the interests of the public, employers, clients, employees, colleagues and the profession. Avoid all conduct or practice that is likely to discredit the profession or deceive the public.
ISSUE public statements only in an objective and truthful manner and only when founded upon knowledge of the facts and competence in the subject matter.
UNDERTAKE assignments only when qualified by education or experience in the specific technical fields involved. Accept responsibility for their continued professional development by acquiring and maintaining competence through continuing education, experience, professional training and keeping current on relevant legal issues.
AVOID deceptive acts that falsify or misrepresent their academic or professional qualifications. Not misrepresent or exaggerate their degree of responsibility in or for the subject matter of prior assignments. Presentations incident to the solicitation of employment shall not misrepresent pertinent facts concerning employers, employees, associates, or past accomplishments with the intent and purpose of enhancing their qualifications and their work.
CONDUCT their professional relations by the highest standards of integrity and avoid compromise of their professional judgment by conflicts of interest. When becoming aware of professional misconduct by a BCSP certificant, take steps to bring that misconduct to the attention of the Board of Certified Safety Professionals.
ACT in a manner free of bias with regard to religion, ethnicity, gender, age, national origin, sexual orientation, or disability.
SEEK opportunities to be of constructive service in civic affairs and work for the advancement of the safety, health and wellbeing of their community and their profession by sharing their knowledge and skills.

Program Evaluation and Continuous Improvement

According to ANSI Z10-2012, an Occupational Health and Safety Management System (OHSMS) is defined as a set of interrelated elements that establish and/or support occupational health and safety policy and objectives. The OHSMS should provide mechanisms to achieve those objectives to continually improve occupational health and safety. The illustration below depicts how the OHSMS requirements can enhance the approach to managing health and safety program activities. The circle in the middle of the diagram shows the OHSMS continuous improvement cycle based on the concept of "Plan-Do-Check-Act."

The management system approach is characterized by its emphasis on continual improvement and systematically eliminating the root causes of mishaps. The processes that drive the implementation of the organizational management system facilitates improved teamwork and operational performance. Establish performance objectives, especially for those issues with the greatest opportunity for safety improvement and risk reduction.

OHSMS objectives should meet "SMART" criteria:
- Specific—Clearly defined desired outcome
- Measurable—Concrete metric for success
- Actionable—Written as a concrete action plan
- Realistic—Practical in its scope
- Time-bounded—A specific timeframe is set

OHSMS evaluation and improvement involves continuous analysis of management leadership and employee involvement, hazard prevention and control, training and education. This may involve periodic review of program operations to evaluate success in meeting the goal and objectives. A comprehensive program audit is needed to evaluate the safety and health management means, methods, and processes, to ensure they are protecting against worksite hazards. The audit determines whether the policies and procedures are implemented as planned and whether they have met the objectives set for the program. This allows for the identification of opportunities for improvement and can inform the strategic planning process.

The success of an OHSMS requires a strategic map that describes major processes and milestones that need to be implemented and maintained to achieve a safe and healthful workplace. This strategy is intended focus on the process rather than on individual tasks. It is common for most sites to have a tendency to focus on the accomplishment of tasks, i.e., to train everyone on a particular concern or topic or implement a new procedure for incident investigations.

Sites that maintain their focus on the larger process are far more successful. They can see the trending issues and thus can make system adjustments as needed. They never lose sight of their intended goals, and tend not to get distracted or allow obstacles to interfere with their mission. The process itself will take care of the task implementation and ensure that the appropriate resources are provided and priorities are set. An organization may use a qualitative or a quantitative evaluation system based on its size, operations, services, and culture.

An essential part of any safety and health system is the correction of hazards that occur despite the overall prevention and control program. For larger sites, documentation is important so that management and employees have a record of the correction.

Many companies use the form that documents the original discovery of a hazard to track its correction. Hazard correction information can be noted on an inspection report next to the hazard description. Employee reports of hazards and reports of accident investigation should provide space for notations about hazard correction.
Frequently, companies will computerize their hazard tracking system which can be as simple as adding a few items to an existing database, such as work order tracking.

Objectives for measuring safety performance:
- Representative forms and procedures
- Information gathering
- Develop safe work practices
- Appropriate feedback based on data
- Documenting safety efforts
- Justify resources
- Stimulating prevention action
- Reinforcing performance improvement

Inputs to the Management review process may include:
- Progress in the reduction of risk;
- Effectiveness of processes to identify, assess, and prioritize risk and system deficiencies;

- Effectiveness in addressing root causes of risks and system deficiencies;
- Input from employees and employee representatives;
- Status of corrective and preventative actions;
- Follow-up actions from OHSMS audits and previous management reviews;
- The extent to which objectives have been met; and
- The performance of the OHSMS relative to expectations, taking into consideration changing circumstances, resource needs, alignment of the business plan and consistency with occupational health and safety policy.

Top management reviews are critical because they have the authority to make the necessary decisions about actions and resources, although it may also be appropriate to include other employee and management levels in the process. To be effective, the review process should ensure the necessary information is available for top management to evaluate the continuing suitability, adequacy, and effectiveness of the OHSMS. Reviews should present results to assist top management with prioritizing OHSMS elements. At the conclusion of the reviews, top management should make decisions, provide direction, and commit resources to implement the decisions.

Performance Problem Characteristics

MOTIVATIONAL ISSUES	ENVIRONMENTAL BARRIERS	SKILL/KNOWLEDGE DEFICIENCY
Individuals not in appropriate job for their training. Individuals not getting clear/timely feedback on performance. Punishment is a management technique. Lack of clarity as to role in unit mission. Good performance is punished. Non-performance is rewarded. Reward system is minimal or no reward for quality performance. Tasks are distasteful.	New equipment, system, or process present. Required support equipment broken or missing from unit. Work facilities inadequate. Barriers to performance Staffing shortages. Work flow unclear. Supply and demand difficulties. Frequent supervisory changes. High Turnover	Individuals observed not performing a task correctly Practice of tasks is non routine or unrealistic. Task requires the application of concepts, rules, and principles. Task is new to job A trend of inadequate training Performance is complex and must be performed without using job aids. Performance is guided, but the guides are poorly written. Performance is poorly defined or described.

Below are some possible solutions to motivational and environmental problems, deficiencies in skills and knowledge, and flawed incentives and policies.

CAUSE	SOLUTIONS
Weak motivation	Information. Job aids. Coaching. Mentoring.
Faulty environment	Job redesign. New tools. Technology.
Absence of skill/knowledge	Training. Information. Job aid. Coaching. Mentoring.
Flawed incentives/policies	New policies. Management development. Supervisory training.

Ten OHSMS Strategies

1). Define safety responsibilities for all levels of the organization, e.g., safety is a line management function.

2). Develop upstream measures, e.g., number of reports of hazards/suggestions, number of committee projects/successes, etc.

3). Align management and supervisors by establishing a shared vision of safety and health goals and objectives vs. production.

4). Implement a process that holds managers and supervisors accountable for visibly being involved, setting the proper example, and leading a positive safety and health culture.

5). Evaluate effectiveness of recognition and disciplinary systems for safety and health.

6). Ensure the safety committee is functioning appropriately, e.g., membership, responsibilities/functions, authority, meeting management skills.

7). Provide multiple paths for employees to bring forward suggestions, concerns, or problems. One mechanism should use the chain of command and ensure no repercussions. Hold supervisors and middle managers accountable for being responsive.

8). Develop a system that tracks and ensures timeliness in hazard correction. Many sites have been successful in building this in with an already existing work order system.

9). Ensure reporting of injuries, first aid cases, and the near misses. Educate employees about the accident pyramid and importance of reporting minor incidents. Prepare management for an initial increase in incidents and a rise in rates. This will occur if underreporting exists in the organization. It will level off, then decline as the system changes take hold.

10). Evaluate and rebuild the incident investigation system as necessary to ensure that investigations are timely, complete, and effective. They should get to the root causes and avoid blaming workers.

Education and Training

Education and training are critical for developing the skills and knowledge of workplace hazards and how employees protect themselves from those hazards. It is important that everyone in the workplace is properly trained. This includes the worker to the supervisors, managers, contractors, and part-time and temporary workers. It is important to distinguish that training is not education. Education is generally measured by tenure: you spent a day in the seminar or four years in college. Training, on the other hand, is measured by what you can do when you've completed it.

- Training delivers the skills to do something rather than just know about something. Training involves practical application of the knowledge and skill.
- Education is all about learning the theory and more importantly, transferring that learning into new or different situations. Traditionally, an education may reinforce knowledge in which that you already have a foundation.

Supervisors and managers should be trained to recognize hazards and understand their responsibilities. The organization should establish a process to:

- Define and assess the OHSMS competence needed for employees and contractors
- Ensure through appropriate education, training, or other methods that employees and contractors are aware of applicable OHSM requirements and competent in their responsibilities.
- Ensure effective access to education and training, and remove barriers to participation.
- Ensure training is provided in a language trainees understand.
- Ensure training is ongoing and timely.
- Ensure trainers are competent to train employees.

Training can help to develop the knowledge and skills needed to understand workplace hazards and safe procedures. It is most effective when integrated into a company's overall training in performance requirements and job practices. The content of a company's training program and the methods of presentation should reflect the needs and characteristics of the particular workforce. Therefore, identification of needs is an important early step in training design. Involving everyone in this process and in the subsequent teaching can be highly effective.

These principles of training should be followed to maximize effectiveness:
- Training needs assessment, will training solve the issue.
- Measurable learning [performance] objectives.
- Trainees should understand the purpose of the training.
- Information should be organized to maximize effectiveness.
- People learn best when they can immediately practice and apply newly acquired knowledge and skills.
- As trainees practice, they should get feedback.
- People learn in different ways, so effective training will incorporate a variety of training methods.

Some examples of health and safety training needed:
- Orientation training for new hires, site workers and contractors
- JSAs, SOPs, and other hazard recognition training
- Training required by OSHA standards: hazard communication, fall protection, operator, electrical, PPE, etc.
- Hazard identification, control and reporting
- Safety inspections
- Accident investigation training
- Emergency drills

Managers and supervisors should also be included in the training plan. Training for managers should emphasize the importance of their role in visibly supporting the safety and health program and setting a good example. Supervisors should receive training in company policies and procedures, as well as hazard detection and control, accident investigation, handling of emergencies, and how to train and reinforce training.

The entire workforce needs periodic refresher training to reinforce OHSMS goals and objectives.

Plan to evaluate the training program when initially designing the training.
If the evaluation is done right, it can identify your program's strengths and weaknesses, and provide a basis for future program changes.
Keeping training records will help ensure that everyone who should get training does. Training documentation may include:
- The targeted audience and learning objective(s)
- Sources used to develop training materials
- Training evaluation methods

- The date location and duration of the training
- Name and description of the course
- Names of trainers delivering the training
- The delivery materials used
- The trainees participating in the training
- The trainees successful completion of the training
- Certification of training and testing

The Adult Learner

In training adults, this focus shifts from the instructor to the participant. And the role of the instructor is not one of lecturer; rather, the instructor becomes a guide and facilitator for the group. This does not mean that the instructor brings no new, unfamiliar information to the group. But even when a lecture is called for, it can be done in a way that makes it an interactive process. It is this interaction that perhaps most characterizes training. Environmental, safety and health trainers are adult participants themselves, so it should be easy to identify with the audience. If trainers would not want to be treated a certain way by their trainers, chances are their participants will not like that approach either.

The following are several characteristics of adult participants that facilitators need to keep in mind as they develop their instructional strategies.
The best training programs take advantage of the following characteristics of adult learners:

- Adults are self-motivated.
- Adults expect to gain information that has immediate application to their lives.
- Adults learn best when they are actively engaged.
- Adult learning activities are most effective when they are designed to allow students to develop both technical knowledge and general skills.
- Adults learn best when they have time to interact, not only with the instructor but also with each other.
- Adults learn best when asked to share each other's personal experiences at work and elsewhere.

There are several guidelines based on the characteristics stated above that will facilitate a successful training session. These guidelines are based on respect for the participants and their experiences. These are also are in recognition of the variety of learning styles in the audience.

The following are the basic principles of how adults learn, which is directly applicable to developing safety and health training programs:

- **Adults are voluntary learners**: Most adults learn because they want to. They learn best when they have decided they need to learn for a particular reason.
- **Adults learn needed information quickly:** Adults need to see that the subject matter and the methods are relevant to their lives and to what they want to learn. They have a right to know why the information is important to them.
- Adults come with a good deal of life experience that needs to be acknowledged: They should be encouraged to share their experiences and knowledge.
- **Adults need to be treated with respect**: They resent an instructor who talks down to them or ignores their ideas and concerns.
- **Adults learn more when they participate in the learning process**: Adults need to be involved and actively participating in class.
- **Adults learn best by doing**: Adults need to "try-on" and practice what they are learning. They will retain more information when they use and practice their knowledge and skills in class.
- **Adults need to know where they are heading**: Learners need "route maps," with clear objectives. Each new piece of information needs to build logically on the last.
- **Adults learn best when new information is reinforced and repeated**: Adults need to hear things more than once. They need time to master new knowledge, skills, and attitudes. They need to have this mastery reinforced at every opportunity.
- **Adults learn better when information is presented in different ways**: They will learn better when an instructor uses a variety of teaching techniques.

The following provides a brief summary of adult learning principles:

1. Focus on "real world" problems.
2. Emphasize how the learning can be applied.
3. Relate the learning to the learner's goal.
4. Allow debate and challenge of ideas.
5. Relate the materials to the learners' experiences.
6. Listen to and respect the opinions of learners.
7. Encourage learners to be resources to you and to each other.
8. Treat learners like adults.

Controlling problem individuals at a meeting is sometimes necessary for a leader. The following list categorizes some of these problem types and a possible method of effectively handling these disruptive individuals. It is important to keep in mind that one or two responses, though they may be perfect examples of a pattern we are discussing, do not make a pattern. In other words, it is not necessary or appropriate to intervene each time a group member manifests a disruptive bit of behavior, only when the behavior becomes repetitive, is having a negative effect on the group, or is becoming irritating to you does it become a pattern. At this point it is desirable to intervene in order to eliminate the behavior. It is important to remember that the *behavior is not the person*. It is only one aspect of the person. When an individual is showing a negative side, it is difficult to see the positive side. You, as a leader, need to reinforce any positive behaviors and attempt to minimize the negative ones.

Trainers should monitor progress in the learning environment and make appropriate adjustments. Consider the following:

- Actively involve participants in the learning process.
- Make participants accountable for learning and participation.
- Design problem-solving activities.
- Create a learner-centered, rather than instructor-centered, learning environment.
- Observe verbal and non-verbal cues from the learner.

The vast majority of students who attend safety and health training sessions are adults who already possess the knowledge, skills, and abilities to work in their current occupations. The objective of safety and health training is to provide additional knowledge, skills, and attitudes to assist workers in recognizing and taking action to correct hazards in their current work environments. Good trainers appreciate the knowledge, skills and experiences that adult participants have possess prior to attending training.

The challenge for trainers that stand up in front of a group, they tend to follow the example of their high school teachers or higher Ed professors. It is very easy to assume the role of a lecturer because that is the standard academic model, the pedagogical model. Trainers should view themselves as "facilitators," helping adults learn.

Training Needs Assessment

Is Training the Solution?

The first activity before entering the instructional system design process is to determine whether there is an instructional need. The application of a needs assessment and needs analysis makes certain that the critical performance requirements of an organization establish the content of training. Training is not the solution for all performance deficiencies. It is neither efficient nor cost effective to produce training without valid justification.

A needs assessment is the process used to identify and document a gap between the desired and actual unit or individual human performance, as well as determine the cause for the gap. Needs assessment can be reactive in identifying deficiencies between what exists and what is required. Needs assessment can also identify potential deficiencies between current and future requirements as a result of changes in threat, policies, organizational structure, leadership development, and equipment.

The needs assessment provides a means to identify the gaps between current results and desired results (a comparison of "what is" with "what should be"). Needs assessment is designed to maximize the use of resources in identifying and resolving performance deficiencies. Training should not be developed or revised unless needs assessment determines that training is the means to resolve the deficiencies and that the needs analysis shows there is a requirement.

Identify the Performance Discrepancy

The beginning point of a needs assessment is a unit or human performance problem. It is necessary to collect, group, and analyze the symptoms of the problem to identify the performance discrepancy. The identification of a problem does not signal the requirement for a training solution, but rather only signals the requirement to continue the needs assessment process. The needs assessment process may include the following: a. Collect, group, and analyze the triggering circumstances, symptoms, or indicators in the problem identification process.

Triggering circumstances or documents may include but are not limited to:
(1) Supervisors comments.
(2) Safety, quality, production reports.
(3) Work Order/Maintenance reports.
(4) Worker comments.
(5) Identification of a new or changed operation.
(6) Introduction of a new piece of equipment.
(7) New Job Description, SOPs, JSA/JHA, or tasks.
(8) Audits, inspections, and evaluations.
(9) Safety reports.
(10) Changes in policy or procedures.
(11) Lessons learned, continuous improvement initiatives.

A systematic problem-solving approach that can support the accomplishment of needs assessment. Begin by raising questions. The answers to these questions can isolate the essence of the performance discrepancy, and later analysis will suggest acceptable solutions. An example of questions to be answered during needs assessment are as follows:
(1) What is the real problem?
(2) What is the extent and gravity of this problem (safety/security/environmental)?
(3) What other symptoms are there that indicate the extent of this problem?
(4) Who is deficient?
(5) When is the problem present?
(6) What impact does this problem have on unit performance?
(7) What is the impact on critical task performance?
(8) What is the impact on unit mission?
(9) Is this problem attributable to a skills/knowledge deficiency?
(10) Is this an environmental or motivational problem?
(11) What is the major cause of this problem?
(12) What are contributing causes to this problem?
(13) What are the constraints that hamper problem identification?

Document the evidence supporting the possible problem. Determine whether doctrine, training, organization, leadership, equipment, or a combination of these is the cause of the performance problem. The needs assessment process may indicate that the problem is motivational or environmental rather than a lack of knowledge or skill. Proceed with a needs analysis only if the environment and motivation issues prove negative and the problem is one of a knowledge or skills deficiency.

Learning Objectives

One product of the analysis phase is a list of tasks that require training. The list of tasks should be arranged in a hierarchy of skills with supporting knowledge and attitudes. In the design phase, use this task list and the task analysis to develop Learning Objectives (LO) for the course. LOs should be stated in terms of what the students must be able to do at the completion of training. Ensure that LOs are developed to fully support all the knowledge, skill, and attitude requirements between the students' entry-level baseline and the mastery level identified for the training program. A LO is a precise statement of the capability or Knowledge, Skill and Ability (KSA) a student is expected to demonstrate, the condition under which the KSA is to be exhibited, and the standard of acceptable performance. Some projects involve the development of new LOs with an existing task list. In this situation, a learning analysis should be conducted to ensure a complete list of KSAs. The goal is to make training realistic and relevant to the work environment[22]. LOs serve several purposes. Some examples are shown below:

1) For instructional developers, the LO will:
   a) Provide a basis for test item development.
   b) Allow for selection of the most appropriate training strategies.
   c) Structure events and activities to support learning.
   d) Supports final selection of appropriate and cost efficient methods
   e) Supports sequencing of training.

2) For students, the LO will:
   a) Direct attention to the important content.
   b) Communicate standard of performance expected following the training.
   c) Serve as a self-check for progress.

There are many terms used that mean the same thing as LOs. Regardless of what they are called, they are all LOs. The following terms are at times used to refer to LOs:

(1) Performance objectives.
(2) Behavioral objectives.
(3) Instructional objectives.
(4) Training objectives.
(5) Criterion objectives.
(6) Knowledge objectives.

---

[22] Department of Defense MIL-HDBK-29612-2A, (2001) "Instructional Systems Development/Systems Approach to Training and Education" (Part 2 OF 5 Parts)

Learning Objectives are written from the perspective of what the *participant* will be able to do in clear and measureable terms.

Unclear: The trainer will train participants to be aware and know about chemicals.

Clear: Given a chemical name and 1 minute using the workstation computer, supervisors should be able to locate the SDS on the intranet server and describe the hazards and controls needed to protect workers.

Observable Action Verbs			
activate	address	adjust	align
analyze	apply	arrange	assemble
assess	assist	associate	build
balance	categorize	breakdown	change
calculate	check	center	cite
classify	clean	choose	combine
compare	complete	close	connect
construct	contrast	compute	copy
count	create	convert	cut
define	demonstrate	critique	design
detect	determine	describe	diagram
differentiate	distinguish	develop	disconnect
display	enumerate	discharge	draw
duplicate	exhibit	drape	evacuate
examine	flush	estimate	file
fill	grasp	explain	formulate
heat	hold	form	group
illustrate	indicate	grind	identify
install	interpret	insert	inspect
lift	list	label	letter
locate	loosen	listen	load
make	manage	manipulate	machine
measure	modify	mount	mark up
name	open	operate	move
organize	outline	perform	order
plan	predict	prepare	place
press	purchase	produce	prescribe
pull	reassemble	push	quote
read	recondition	rebuild	recall
recite	repack	record	reiterate
remove	reply	repair	repeat
replace	serve	select	respond
restate	signal	service	separate
sequence	speak	sketch	set
show	subdivide	specify	slide
solve	trace	synthesize	state
tap	tune	tighten	tabulate
touch	utilize	transcribe	transfer

Objectives must be **measurable** and **observable.** They should have specific verbs (action words). They should describe something the trainer can see participants do or hear them say. Avoid using words in objectives that are difficult or impossible to measure.

Appropriate Words (Observable - Measurable Behavior)		Inappropriate Words (Not Observable - Non-measurable Behavior)	
write	explain	accept	appreciate
classify	list	be aware of	believe
calculate	select	remember	comprehend
prepare	apply	regard	know
operate	choose	be familiar with	understand
define	construct	consider	discern
describe	complete	grasp	ascertain
demonstrate		value	

Learning Objectives have three parts: 1) a behavior, 2) a condition, and 3) a standard. Before starting to develop LOs, become thoroughly familiar with each part of a LO. Familiarity with the different parts will enable the development of better LOs, and thus, better training. LOs should be worded carefully so that all readers or listeners have the same understanding.

1) **_Behavior._** The behavior part of the LO states what a student will do to demonstrate that he/she learned a specific knowledge, skill, or attitude. A behavior is defined as a KSA that is observable and measurable. When stating the behavior in a LO, use action verbs to reduce ambiguity. Action verbs are observable and measurable while ambiguous verbs are not.

2) **_Condition_**. A thorough understanding of the conditions will help to develop effective LOs. A condition identifies the situation under which a student is expected to demonstrate a behavior. A properly prepared LO clearly states the limits or conditions of student performance.
   a) When determining the conditions for the LOs, consider that:
      i) Conditions should specify the objects, events, human behavior, words, or symbols, which will be presented to the students.
      ii) Conditions under which the training is performed should be the same as the actual job conditions, if possible.

iii) Conditions should be written with particular care to include, in sufficient detail, and safety, health & environmental (SH&E) related conditions which apply to the action being developed into a LO.

b) Condition statements can normally be derived from the task analysis data. The following are some examples of conditions:

i) "Given the diameter of a sphere and the formula, . . ."

ii) "Using a dosimeter and schematic diagram, . . ."

iii) "Without reference, . . ."

iv) "Given an SCBA and Level A chemical protective suit…."

v) "Under conditions of total darkness, . . ."

3) **_Standard._** The final part of a well prepared LO is a clearly stated standard of performance. The student's performance will result in an output, the quantity or quality of which is the standard of performance. If no standards were identified in the task analysis data that was previously collected, set standards based on other sources such as experience or similar tasks. A standard defines the criteria for acceptable performance by the student. It is stated in terms such as completeness, accuracy requirements, time constraints, performance rates, and qualitative requirements. It identifies the proficiency the students must achieve when they perform the behavior under the specified conditions. Without a standard, it is impossible to determine when the students have achieved the LO.

Documentation

Training providers should maintain records listing the dates courses were presented, the names of the individual course attendees, the names of those students successfully completing each course, and the number of training certificates issued to each successful student. These records should be maintained for a minimum of five years after the date an individual participated in a training program offered by the training provider. These records should be available and provided upon the student's request or as mandated by law. The documentation should include:

a. Participant sign-in sheet/Training roster.

b. Course title and training outline.

c. Course date and materials.

d. Statement or proof that the student has successfully completed the training.

e. Name and address of the training provider (if appropriate).

It is essential to document all training for several reasons:

1)   Training records must be maintained to document that employees have received the proper training to perform their jobs safely.

2)   When inspectors visit a company, they usually review training records to determine if training requirements have been met.

3)   When accurate records are not kept, training has to be repeated to document skills and knowledge.

4)   Proper documentation may be required before employees can work at certain sites or perform certain jobs.

5)   Training records keep trainers organized and assist with continuous improvement efforts.

Usually, documentation is maintained in two types of files. One type of file maintains the files under the heading of the workshop title and is located in the Training Department. The other file lists the workshops attended by each employee; it is often kept in the Human Resources Department.

Criteria for Accepted Practices in Safety, Health and Environmental Training.[23]

The Committee Z490 on Criteria for Accepted Practices in Safety, Health and Environmental Training was accredited by the American National Standards Institute (ANSI) on April 1, 1998 based on the recognized need for improvement in safety, health, and environmental training. The American Society of Safety Professionals (ASSP) is the Secretariat for the Z490 National Standard Committee.

The Z490 standard embraces the concept that quality training is necessary to ensure that workers and safety, health, and environmental professionals have the knowledge, skills, and abilities necessary to protect themselves and others in the workplace.

Safety, health, and environmental training is an important element of an effective overall safety, health, and environmental program. Historically, safety, health, and environmental training has been specifically addressed by only a few regulations with limited scope, such as asbestos, hazard communication, and storm water management. The regulations usually specify the technical topics to be covered in a training course, but do not stipulate how to adequately design, develop, deliver, and evaluate training.

This Z490 Standard comprehensively covers the aspects of training, including training development, delivery, evaluation, and management of training and training programs. The criteria were developed by combining accepted practices in the training industry with those in the safety, health, and environmental industries and it is intended to apply universally to training programs.

Governmental regulations specify mandatory requirements for various safety, health, and environmental training. Likewise, the training program may be embedded in a larger safety, human resources, or other organizational structure. As a broad-based voluntary consensus standard, the Z490 complements the regulations and organizational policies. Like all voluntary or consensus standards, however, compliance with this Standard does not ensure compliance with governmental regulations or organizational policies, or vice versa.

---

[23] ANSI/ASSE Z490.1 (2009) American National Standard, Criteria for Accepted Practices in Safety, Health and Environmental Training.

Overview of the ASSP/ANSI Z490.1 Standard

1. Scope, Purpose, and Application
2. Definitions
3. Training Program Administration and Management
   - Resource Management and Administration
   - Program Evaluation
4. Training Development
   - Needs Assessment
   - Learning Objectives and Prerequisites
   - Course Design
   - Evaluation Strategy
   - Criteria for Completion
   - Continuous Improvement
5. Training Delivery
   - Trainer Criteria
   - Training Delivery Methods and Materials
6. Training Evaluation
   - General Criteria
   - Evaluation Approaches
   - Continuous Improvement
7. Documentation and Record Keeping
   - Systems and Procedure
   - Records
   - Record Confidentiality and Availability
   - Issuing Certificates

Annex A References
Annex B Training Course Development Guidelines
Annex C Safety, Health and Environmental Trainer's Checklist

Domain 4: Quiz 1 Questions

1) The **best** way to deal with minor infractions of work or safety rules?
   A) Oral reprimand.
   B) Written reprimand.
   C) Ignore it.
   D) Suspension.

2) The simplest and **most** effective way to display data to get an instant picture is the use of the?
   A) Line chart.
   B) Bar chart.
   C) Pie chart.
   D) Area chart.

3) According to contemporary motivation theory, the strongest motivator is:
   A) Fear of a boss.
   B) Status.
   C) Recognition of achievement.
   D) Pay.

4) Which of the following responsibilities is not assigned to the National Institute for Occupational Safety and Health (NIOSH)?
   A) Research and identification of occupational safety/health hazards.
   B) Recommending changes to safety/health regulations.
   C) Training of safety/health personnel.
   D) Enforcement of occupational safety/public health standards within the regulated community.

5) Workplace monitoring, employee exposure and medical records must be retained for how long?
   A) 30 years.
   B) Duration of employment plus 30 years.
   C) 5 years.
   D) Duration of employment plus 5 years.

6) The medical questionnaire that is required when you place an employee in your respiratory protection must be evaluated by?
   A) The industrial hygienist.
   B) The safety director.
   C) A licensed health care professional.
   D) Any supervisor.

7) Under which of the following categories would a noise-induced hearing loss be recorded on the OSHA 300 Log?
   A) Disorders due to skin disorder.
   B) Disorders due to injury.
   C) Disorders due to poisoning.
   D) Hearing loss.

8) OSHA requires businesses, both big and small, to report work-related fatalities within eight hours to the nearest OSHA Area Office. What mishaps would require reporting within twenty-four hours?
   A) The injury of an employee that required medical treatment because of a work-related incident.
   B) The in-patient hospitalization of one or more employees because of a work-related incident.
   C) The injury of three or more employees that requires hospitalization or involves traumatic amputation or broken bones because of a work-related incident.
   D) The transport of five or more workers to the hospital because of a work-related incident.

9) Safety, Environmental and Health performance is best presented to upper management in terms of
   A) Lost Workday Incident Rate.
   B) Total fatalities.
   C) Total lost time.
   D) Cost relationships.

10) The use of the term "Accident Proneness" has received considerable attention within the safety community. Current thinking follows which of the following basic theories?
- A) Accident proneness is a fact of life, we must deal with it but we don't have to like it.
- B) Accident proneness should be identified or discounted early in the mishap investigation process.
- C) Accident prone individuals account for 10% of the work force and about 30% of all accidental loss.
- D) Accident proneness is a concept that has no validity in accident prevention work.

11) In the United States what is the major cause of on-the-job injuries?
- A) Motor vehicle accidents.
- B) Falls.
- C) Fire.
- D) Not using PPE.

12) Which of the following techniques is least likely to establish continuous influence on the line manager or supervisor's safety accountability?
- A) Charge accidents to departments.
- B) Put safety in supervisor's appraisal.
- C) Have safety affect supervisor's income.
- D) Require annual safety training for supervisors.

13) Often when interviewing witnesses to an accident or participants in the event, investigators find themselves talking to a hostile and very defensive person. Which of the following methods would most likely result in an honest and truthful statement from these interviewees.
- A) Inform these people that you are going to write everything down and file it, so they better tell the truth.
- B) Tell them the information will only be used for accident prevention purposes and no disciplinary actions will result from your investigation.
- C) Inform the person that you would appreciate it if they would tell you the truth since it will help your position with the company and shouldn't affect them.
- D) Tell them that you are supposed to inform them of their rights, but you are not going to, so they have nothing to fear because anything they say cannot be used against them.

14) Which of the following best describes the legal premise of "chain of custody"?
   A) Secure storage.
   B) Documentation of possession.
   C) Ownership.
   D) Personal knowledge.

15) Effective hazard communication programs for workers using chemicals require:
   A) GHS training, labels, chemical hazard analysis, and Safety Data Sheets.
   B) Safety Data Sheets, chemical inventories, audits, and training.
   C) Bi lingual labels, chemical hazard analysis, chemical inventories, and GHS training.
   D) Hazard classifications, Safety Data Sheets, labels, and training.

16) Who provides the required placards when shipping hazardous material?
   A) The driver.
   B) The carrier.
   C) The shipper.
   D) The manufacturer.

17) The ANSI Z10 is a management system standard compatible and harmonized with quality (ISO 9000 series) and environmental management systems (ISO 14000 series). Which of the following best describes these standards?
   A) Specification standards.
   B) Compliance standards.
   C) Performance standards.
   D) Regulatory standards.

18) The Federal Motor Carrier Safety Administration (FMCSA) is primarily responsible for:
   A)   Research and development for motor carrier safety design.
   B)   Enforcement of motor carrier safety regulations for over the road drivers.
   C)   Outreach and training for hazardous materials shipments.
   D)   Approval of motor carrier drivers and vehicles.

19). Which scenario is **least likely** to use written tests to evaluate one's knowledge of the training objectives?
  A) An ad hoc safety discussion with a work crew.
  B) The training involves a certification process.
  C) Documented effectiveness of the training is required.
  D) The risk of not mastering the training objectives include severe injury, death or financial loss.

20). Which of the following is true concerning the training of personnel who erect and dismantle scaffolding?
  A) Training must be done under the supervision of a certified training instructor.
  B) A competent person must perform the training.
  C) Training is not, and never being required.
  D) Training is a good idea and would ensure safety, but is not required by OSHA.

21). On multi-employer work sites, what is the best method for one employer to inform the other employers about new SDS's?
  A) Develop a system for the general contractor and subcontractors to share SDS's.
  B) The general contractor is responsible.
  C) The superintendent should see that everyone is informed.
  D) Everyone should be responsible for their own.

22). Asbestos training is required to include which of the following?
  A) PPE Selection.
  B) Conducting a negative exposure assessment.
  C) Retention of medical records.
  D) Methods to recognize asbestos.

23). During the planning stage of a Construction Health & Safety Training Program which of the following is the most important consideration?
  A) Training Objectives.
  B) Training Methods.
  C) Instructor Qualifications.
  D) Training Program Content.

24). During a training class, a lesson plan requires that students be able to recall certain facts about personal protective equipment. Which of the following would be true concerning the agencies in the United States that test and approve respiratory protection equipment?

    A) NIOSH
    B) OSHA
    C) NHTSA
    D) DOT

25). Job site safety training is critical part of a safety program. Which of the following statements is most true?

    A) While comprehensive, pre-assignment training covering company assigned topics is necessary, all workers perform best when allowed to self-study training materials.
    B) While comprehensive, pre-assignment training covering regulatory required topics is necessary, on the job experience is the best "trainer." Until workers make their own mistakes, they won't really learn.
    C) Comprehensive, pre-assignment training covering all needed topics and information is the best method of ensuring employees are trained and qualified to perform their tasks safely.
    D) While comprehensive, pre-assignment training covering regulatory required topics is necessary, short, single topic tailgate meetings are very effective.

Domain 4: Quiz 1 Answers

1) Answer A:

Progressive companies believe the proper way to deal with minor rule infractions is to issue a oral reprimand for the first offense. Progressive discipline is then administered for additional violations.

2) Answer B:

The recommended use of the bar chart is to illustrate comparisons of volume over time

3) Answer C:

Current theory holds that recognition of achievement is the single most important motivator.

4) Answer D:

The National Institute for Occupational Safety and Health (NIOSH) is administratively located within the Center for Disease Control (CDC) who functions as a member of the Public Health Service (PHS) which reports to the Department of Health and Human Services (HHS). NIOSH was originally founded within the Department of Health, Education, and Welfare, which is now HHS, under the provisions of the OSHAct. It has prime responsibility for research to eliminate occupational health and safety hazards. NIOSH has the responsibility to identify hazards and recommend changes in the regulations. It performs testing and certification of workers personal protective equipment, mainly respirators. NIOSH has a very active training grant program that supports university training throughout the country and conducts excellent courses at regional centers. NIOSH also does workplace investigations under 42 CFR Part 85, largely to conduct epidemiological methods research and studies. NIOSH does not provide enforcement actions.

5) Answer B:

OSHA 1910.20, Access to employee exposure and medical records, requires that medical records, which includes workplace monitoring records, be kept for the duration of employment plus 30 years. There is one exception to the 30-year requirement that affects construction employers. The medical records of employees who have worked for less than one year of the employer need not be retained beyond the term of employment if they are provided to the employee upon termination of employment.

6)   Answer C:

1910.134(e)(2)(i) The employer shall identify a physician or other licensed health care professional (PLHCP) to perform medical evaluations using a medical questionnaire or an initial medical examination that obtains the same information as the medical questionnaire.

7)   Answer D:

Recordable occupational illnesses on the OSHA 300 log are categorized as follows:

- Injury
- Skin disorder
- Respiratory conditions
- Poisoning
- Hearing loss
- All other illnesses

8)   Answer B:

The OSHA requirements for reporting fatalities or multiple hospitalization mishaps are contained in 1904.8 which states Employers have to report the following events to OSHA:
- All work-related fatalities
- All work-related in-patient hospitalizations of one or more employees
- All work-related amputations
- All work-related losses of an eye

Employers must report work-related fatalities within **8 hours of finding out about it.** For any in-patient hospitalization, amputation, or eye loss **employers must report the incident within 24 hours of learning about it.**

Only fatalities occurring within 30 days of the work-related incident must be reported to OSHA. Further, for an inpatient hospitalization, amputation or loss of an eye, then incidents must be reported to OSHA only if they occur within 24 hours of the work-related incident. Employers have three options for reporting the event:

- By telephone to the nearest OSHA Area Office during normal business hours.
- By telephone to the 24-hour OSHA hotline (1-800-321-OSHA or 1-800-321-6742).

OSHA is developing a new means of reporting events electronically, which will be released soon and accessible on OSHA's website.
Retrieved 5/28/2015 https://www.osha.gov/recordkeeping2014/reporting.html
OSHA Fact sheet retrieved 5/28/2015
https://www.osha.gov/recordkeeping2014/OSHA3745.pdf

9) Answer D:

Most experts agree that depicting the bottom line cost will have the greatest impact on upper level management. This may be done by comparing losses to budgets or future estimated cost impacts and how they will impact unit costs.

10) Answer D:

Several methods of securing line accountability for safety are widely accepted within the safety community. Current thinking within the safety community follows the belief that accident proneness is not a proven scientific fact, but rather an unfounded hypothesis designed to explain the behavior of humans. The theory is rejected in virtually all safety work. Training and education should be part of professional development to enhance skills and knowledge, however, the other answer choices are consequences more directly related to accountability.

11) Answer A:

Motor vehicle accidents are the largest cause of industrial injuries in the United States.

12)   Answer D:

Current thinking within the safety community would support the contention that all of the actions listed will make line supervision take notice. However, it is also believed that a combination of efforts is required to maintain accountability. Most progressive accident prevention efforts use some combination of these techniques or variations thereof.

13)   Answer B:

Dealing with hostile, belligerent or dishonest witnesses or participants, is a way of life for accident investigators. There are many theories about obtaining frank, candid and honest statements from these people. However, it is generally accepted that the most effective way is to explain that your investigation is for accident prevention purposes only and cannot be used for any type of disciplinary action. This tends to set the person at ease and usually will result in the long run in more open and honest responses about the mishap. However, you must be sure that you are telling the truth about the purposes of your report. Often statements made in safety investigations wind up in personnel files or personnel action documents. You must ensure that your report is, as you said, only going to be used for accident prevention purposes. Do not provide false guarantees, which means you must develop a policy concerning safety investigation prior to the need!

14)   Answer B:

Often if evidence is to be used in a court of law the chain of custody must be documented. The chain of custody is simply a documented explanation of where the evidence was obtained and where it has been since that time. The evidence must have been secured from tampering or change. The court must be assured through the chain of custody that the evidence is unchanged or changes can be explained.

15)   Answer D:

The OSHA Hazard Communication Standard (HCS) is now aligned with the Globally Harmonized System of Classification and Labeling of Chemicals (GHS). In order to ensure chemical safety in the workplace, information about the identities and hazards of the chemicals must be available and understandable to workers. OSHA's Hazard Communication Standard (HCS) requires the development and dissemination of such information:

- Chemical manufacturers and importers are required to evaluate the hazards of the chemicals they produce or import, and prepare labels and safety data sheets to convey the hazard information to their downstream customers;
- All employers with hazardous chemicals in their workplaces must have labels and safety data sheets for their exposed workers, and train them to handle the chemicals appropriately.

An effective Hazard Communication program shall include:

Hazard classification: Provides specific criteria for classification of health and physical hazards, as well as classification of mixtures.

Labels: Chemical manufacturers and importers are required to provide a label that includes a harmonized signal word, pictogram, and hazard statement for each hazard class and category. Precautionary statements must also be provided.

Safety Data Sheets: Specified 16-section format.

Information and training: Employers are required to train workers on the chemical labels elements and safety data sheets.

16) Answer C:

According to DOT regulations in 49 CFR Part 397, the shipper must:

- transport the products by truck, railroad, ship or airplane;
- determine the product's proper shipping name, hazard class, identification number, correct packaging, correct placard, and correct tables and markings;
- package the materials, label and mark the packages, prepare the shipping paper and **supply the placards**; and
- certify on the shipping paper that he properly complied with the rules for shipment.

17) Answer C:

The drafters of these standards set out to ensure that it could be easily integrated into any management systems an organization has in place. This flexibility is characteristic of a Performance Oriented Standard. Z10 adopts from and is in harmony with the International Labor Organization's Guidelines on Occupational health and Safety Management Systems, ILO-OSH 2001.

18) Answer B:

The Federal Motor Carrier Safety Administration (FMCSA) was established within the Department of Transportation on January 1, 2000, pursuant to the Motor Carrier Safety Improvement Act of 1999 (49 U.S.C. 113). Formerly a part of the Federal Highway Administration, the Federal Motor Carrier Safety Administration's primary mission is to prevent commercial motor vehicle-related fatalities and injuries. Activities of the Administration contribute to ensuring safety in motor carrier operations through strong enforcement of safety regulations; targeting high-risk carriers and commercial motor vehicle drivers; improving safety information systems and commercial motor vehicle technologies; strengthening commercial motor vehicle equipment and operating standards; and increasing safety awareness. To accomplish these activities, the Administration works with Federal, State, and local enforcement agencies, the motor carrier industry, labor safety interest groups, and others.

19) Answer A:

In safety and health training, a knowledge or proficiency tests or evaluations are highly recommended in all the following:
- The training involves a certification or qualification process
- The organizational culture supports its use
- The effectiveness of the training may be questioned
- The risk of not mastering the objectives include injury, death or severe financial loss
- Qualitative and quantitative data are needed pertaining to training and/or safety and health issues

20) Answer B:

OSHA requires a competent person to provide training on the nature of fall hazards, the correct procedures for erection, maintenance and disassembly, the proper use, placement and care in handling, etc. Additionally, all erection and disassembly must be done under the supervision of a competent person.

21) Answer A:

Develop a system for the general contractor and subcontractors to share the SDS's.

22)   Answer D:

Employers must provide a free training program for all employees who are likely to be exposed in excess of a PEL and for all employees performing *Class I* through *IV* asbestos operations. Employees must be trained prior to or at initial assignment and at least annually thereafter. Training courses must be easily understandable and include the following information:

- Ways to recognize asbestos.
- Adverse health effects of asbestos exposure.
- Relationship between smoking and asbestos in causing lung cancer.
- Operations that could result in asbestos exposure and the importance of protective controls to minimize exposure.
- Purpose, proper use, fitting instruction, and limitations of respirators.
- Appropriate work practices for performing asbestos jobs.
- Medical surveillance program requirements.
- Contents of the standard.
- Names, addresses, and phone numbers of public health organizations that provide information and materials or conduct smoking cessation programs.
- Sign and label requirements and the meaning of their legends.
- Written materials relating to employee training and self help smoking cessation programs at no cost to employees.

Also, the following additional training requirements apply depending on the work class involved:

- For *Class I* operations and for *Class II* operations that require the use of critical barriers (or equivalent isolation methods) and/or negative pressure enclosures, training must be equivalent in curriculum, method, and length to the EPA Model Accreditation Plan (MAP) asbestos abatement worker training (see 40 CFR Part 763, Subpart E, Appendix C).
- For employees performing *Class II* operations involving one generic category of building materials containing asbestos (e.g., roofing, flooring, or siding materials or transite panels), training may be covered in an 8-hour course that includes hands-on experience.
- For *Class III* operations, training must be equivalent in curriculum and method to the 16-hour *Operations and Maintenance* course developed by EPA for maintenance and custodial workers whose work disturbs ACM (see 40 CFR Part 763.92). The course must include hands-on training on proper respirator use and work practices.

- For *Class IV* operations, training must be equivalent in curriculum and method to EPA awareness training (see 29 CFR Part1926.1101 for more information). Training must focus on the locations of ACM or PACM and the ways to recognize damage and deterioration and avoid exposure. The course must be at least 2 hours in length.

On all construction sites with asbestos operations, employers must designate a *competent person*—one who can identify asbestos hazards in the workplace and has the authority to correct them. This person must be qualified and authorized to ensure worker safety and health as required by *Subpart C, General Safety and Health Provisions for Construction* (29 CFR Part 1926.20). Under these requirements for safety and health prevention programs, the *competent person* must frequently inspect job sites, materials, and equipment. The *competent person* must attend a comprehensive training course for contractors and supervisors certified by the U.S. Environmental Protection Agency (EPA) or a state approved training provider, or a complete a course that is equivalent in length and content. For *Class III and IV* asbestos work, training must include a course equivalent in length, stringency, and content to the 16-hour *Operations and Maintenance* course developed by EPA for maintenance and custodial workers. For more specific information, see 40 CFR Part 763.92(a)(2).

23) Answer A:

The establishment of Training Objectives is the key to good planning. No other single element has the ability to allow the training program to succeed.

24) Answer A:

Within the United States both NIOSH test and approve respiratory protection.

25) Answer D:

Safety training is a crucial part of a comprehensive safety program. There are many topics that regulations require training to be accomplished prior to job assignment. Industry has recognized that ongoing training provided for short periods of time (less than an hour), covering single topics is a very effective method to training workers. The key to safety training is to provide workers with information to prevent accidents and injuries.

Domain 4: Quiz 2 Questions

1). Training mandated by the Hazard Communication Standard is accomplished to allow employees to become familiar with the hazards of chemicals in the workplace and protective measures. Which of the following statements is most correct concerning HazCom training done by a commercial training company?
   - A) OSHA will cite the commercial training company for any training deficiencies
   - B) OSHA will cite the employer for any training deficiencies
   - C) OSHA will cite both the employer and the training company for any training deficiencies
   - D) OSHA will cite the training company only if it has been licensed and approved by OSHA

2). Your company has hired a new worker who was qualified as a powered truck operator at her previous company. What is the training required to get this person qualified as a power truck operator in your company?
   - A) Send to a formal school
   - B) Accept the other company's qualification
   - C) Have the employee attend your company's initial training program
   - D) Ensure the operator has the knowledge and skills required to operate the power trucks, including your company's procedures.

3). The primary purpose for using On-the-Job training is:
   - A) It is cost effective
   - B) More than one person can be trained at a time
   - C) Requires the minimum amount of time for total training
   - D) Allows the worker to produce during the training period

4). A needs assessment does all the following except:
   - A) Identifies the type of training required
   - B) Identifies the problem or need before designing a solution
   - C) Saves time and money by ensuring that solutions effectively address the problems they are intended to solve
   - D) Identifies factors that will impact the training before its development

5). Which **best** describes the purpose of post training testing?
   A) To compare weak performers to strong performers.
   B) To identify workers who have "attitude" problems.
   C) To identify improvements in the training program and measure the learner's knowledge, skill or attitude.
   D) To document the training event for future audits.

6). Which of the following is the ***best indicator*** of training effectiveness?
   A) Favorable Student Critiques
   B) Correct Student Response to Questions
   C) Increase in effectiveness of Job Performance
   D) Testing meets expected norms

7). Verbs or actions words used in learning objectives must be as specific as possible. The behavior must be observable and measurable. Which of the following verbs **does not** meet this criterion?
   A) Understand
   B) Identify
   C) Troubleshoot
   D) Enter data

8). Employee training records maintained for bloodborne pathogens must be retained for:
   A) 3 years from the date of training
   B) Duration of employment plus 3 years
   C) 5 years from the date of training
   D) Duration of employment plus 5 years

9). The **primary** purpose of safety committee is:
   A) Pass the responsibility to employees
   B) Improve communication to/from management and employees
   C) Allow employees the voice they need
   D) Show OSHA the company cares

10). According to the OSHA Hazard Communication Standard which of the following would **not** require employers to provide employees training on the hazardous chemicals in the workplace?
    A) Initial assignment
    B) Resupply of chemicals
    C) Change in job assignment with new chemicals
    D) New chemical hazard in the work environment

11). After safety training is completed, there are many ways to continue to encourage safety at the job site. The **best** includes:
    A) Setting a good example, encouraging safe behavior, follow up on complaints and hazard reports
    B) Setting a good example, strictly enforcing all safety requirements, follow up on complaints and hazard reports
    C) Encouraging safe behavior, require persons that report problems to fix them, setting a good example
    D) Getting worker to clearly document their safety concerns, strictly enforcing all safety requirements, performing surprise checks of equipment

12). The **primary** purpose of safety education and training is:
    A) To prepare for testing
    B) To meet regulatory requirements
    C) To minimize insurance premiums
    D) To impart knowledge and ability

13). Safety training is **best** delivered:
    A) As an integrated part of all other training
    B) By the front line supervisor
    C) By a contracted trainer
    D) By co-workers

14). When is training **least** appropriate:
    A) At the beginning of shift
    B) After an incident
    C) After a recordable injury
    D) At end of work shift

15). Which of the following **is not** a communication barrier?
    A) Bias
    B) Mood
    C) Negative reinforcement
    D) Nonverbal actions that conflict with the training subject

16). Successful adult training can be measured by all of the following except?
    A) Demonstrate the application
    B) Show a tape of a previous experience
    C) Let the trainee practice the new skill
    D) Discuss how the new skills can be applied

17). Who is in the best position to provide effective safety training of industrial work groups?
    A) Supervisors
    B) Senior Management
    C) CHSTs
    D) Training Professionals

18). Which of the following is not an expected outcome of group training?
    A) Gain skills
    B) Share ideas
    C) Evaluate information
    D) Become actively involved in the planning and implementation of company policy

19). During Health and Safety communications with workers, the main objective is to?
    A) Teach workers to understand what is being said
    B) Provide a vehicle for suggestions
    C) Teach workers to write and read well
    D) Provide a safety message that will be understood and accepted by the workers

20). A lesson plan is primarily designed to?
    A) Be provided as a training class handout.
    B) Provide the learners with the course objectives.
    C) Provide standardized guidance for the training session.
    D) Review prior to the beginning of the training session.

21). Communication is defined as?
   A) Sharing information and/or ideas with others and being understood
   B) Sharing information and/or ideas with others and gaining approval
   C) Sharing opinions and/or ideas with others and being understood
   D) Sharing opinions and/or ideas with others and gaining approval

22). During a training session, often you will attempt to change the way your audience views their procedures or actions. A primary way to help facilitate change is to:
   A) Allow everyone to express their point of view
   B) Follow the lesson plan without interruptions
   C) Allow limited questions at the end of the presentation
   D) Point out how the change will affect the workplace

23). What defines successful communications?
   A) Sender and message
   B) Sender and receiver
   C) Message and receiver
   D) Sender, message and receiver

24). Communications has many forms, which is the most effective in the workplace?
   A) Face to face group lecture
   B) Face to face group two-way communications
   C) Face to face individual two-way communications
   D) Written individual two-way communications

25). One-way communications have several short falls. Which of the following is not a short fall?
   A) The information will be transmitted correctly
   B) Information flows in only one direction
   C) Lack of feedback
   D) Receiver may not understand the message

Domain 4: Quiz 2 Answers

1) **Answer B:**

The following information was extracted from the Hazard Communication Standard "QUIP" published by OSHA. In response to a request for clarification OSHA stated "If it is determined that an employee has not received training or is not adequately trained, the current employer will be held responsible regardless of who provided the training to the employee. An employer, therefore, has a responsibility to evaluate an employee's level of knowledge with regard to the training and information requirements of the standard, and the employer's own hazard communication program, including previous training the employee may have received."

2) **Answer D:**

CFR1910.178, Powered Industrial Trucks, requires anyone changing equipment or workplace location to meet the requirements outlined in the Refresher Training requirements (para 1910.178 (l)(4)). Only employees that are trained and authorized should operate industrial powered trucks.

3) **Answer D:**

According to the NSC, OJT or JIT is widely used because it allows the worker to produce during the training period. The primary instruction is the demonstration or demonstration-performance method of training.

4) **Answer A:**

According to the NSC, a needs assessment helps to:
- Distinguishes between training and non-training needs
- Identifies the problem or need before designing a solution
- Saves time and money by ensuring that solutions effectively address the problems they are intended to solve
- Identifies factors that will impact the training before its development

After the first step in the training process which is the needs assessment, training goals are developed and during that process you will determine what knowledge the trainee needs to know to eliminate the problem. Remember, if you want them to tell time, then teach them how to tell time, not how to build a watch.

5)   Answer C:

In the practice of Safety and Health, training is often offered as a universal solution. However, safety and health training should be targeted to real problems. Training should only be recommended as the solution to problems where increased knowledge or skill is needed or where required by directive. There are two objectives to post training testing. First, to see if the student has gained skill or knowledge in the subject area. Second, to assist the developer and instructor in evaluating the effectiveness of instruction. For example, if a significant percentage of the students in an average class cannot perform up to the specifications outlined in the lesson plans, then the instruction is simply not working. The problem could be the atmosphere, the instructional method, instruction techniques, the instructor, training material, etc. In any event, changes are in order. Effective training is a complex task, in which evaluation of the instruction is often overlooked. One thing that cannot be corrected by training is "poor worker attitude". This is often a complaint against the training staff is that the attitude hasn't changed, but generally that is the responsibility of the supervisor.

6)   Answer C:

Job performance is the most effective and final measure of any training program and the training should be designed to correct skill deficiencies. Testing is highly recommended when the effectiveness of the training may be questioned.

7)   Answer A:

Some words that should be avoided when writing learning objectives are; know, understand, appreciate, learn, cover, study. It is almost impossible to determine if the student has accomplished those objectives. Some example preferred words are; explain, classify compare, calculate, demonstrate, operate, measure, troubleshoot, analyze, develop, plan.

8)   Answer A:

Employee training records maintained under the provisions of 1910.1030,

Bloodborne Pathogens, must be retained for three year from the date on which the training occurred.

9)   Answer B:
Safety committees are not a 'silver bullet' that will fix safety concerns. They are a good method for raising issues for consideration, for discussing potential solutions, and for galvanizing personnel during implementing improvements. The way the most successful committees do these things is through open and candid communication between organizational leaders from both management and the front line.

10)   Answer B:

According to the OSHA Hazard Communication Standard (29 CFR 1926.59) employers shall provide employees with information and training on hazardous chemicals in their work area:
- at time of initial assignment
- if transferred to a new assignment with new chemical hazards
- when a new chemical hazard is introduced into the work place

11)   Answer A:

Research has shown that a positive environment encourages better safety by workers than an environment based strictly on enforcement. Enforcement is an important aspect of a safety program, but positive encouragement before enforcement is best. It is crucial to set a positive example as the supervisor by following **all** safety requirements. The supervisor needs to follow up on all complaints and hazard reports

12)   Answer D:

Training is provided to impart knowledge and ability. In the case of safety training, the primary objective is to impart knowledge and ability to allow a worker to prevent injuries and accidents.

13)   Answer B:

Safety training is best delivered by the front-line supervisor.

14) Answer D:

Training is least effective and appropriate at the end of the work shift.

15) Answer C:

Communication barriers consist of:
- Knowledge – the trainee already thinks the know all that is needed
- Bias – people's attitude may cause them to tune out the information
- Mood – does something keep the individual from hearing the information
- Nonverbal actions – do you say one thing while doing something counter

16) Answer B:

Adults want satisfactory answers to the following questions to accept and apply learning.
1. Why is it important?
2. How can I apply it?
3. How does it work?
4. What do I need to know?

17) Answer A:

Supervisors are in the best position to provide realistic and effective training for industrial workers. They have detailed knowledge of work processes and control workflow.

18) Answer A:

Group techniques encourage participation from a selected audience. These methods allow trainees to share ideas, evaluate information and become actively involved in the planning and implementation of company policy. Group training is helpful when you need to transfer specific information to a group of people who need to know the same information.

19)   Answer D:

The bottom line in any training or education effort is to provide a message that will be understood and acted on by the workers.

20)   Answer C:

Effective training calls for the use of standardized training. This can be greatly enhanced by using lesson plans. A lesson plan is designed to insure the trainer:
- presents the material in the proper order
- does not omit essential material
- conducts the training on the proper timetable
- places proper emphasis on items to be covered
- provides for student participation
- has confidence in the presentation

21)   Answer A:

According to the NSC, communications is defined as "sharing information and/or ideas with others and being understood".

22)   Answer A:

During any training situation where you are attempting to change habits or procedures, the trainee will have questions as to why it is necessary and is your recommended way the best way. When you allow the trainee to share ideas, evaluate the material and become involved will increase their acceptance of the material.

23)   Answer D:

Communications consists of three basic elements: the sender, the message and the receiver. When you are communicating, whether orally or in writing, always provide for feedback. This is the only way to ensure that the message got through.

24)   Answer C:

Two-way, face-to-face communications is the best way to convey messages on the job.

25)   Answer A:

This type of communications has several problems:
- Information only flows in one direction.
- The lack of feedback means the sender will not know if the message has been received and/or understood. This is the major drawback to one-way communications.
- The receiver may not understand the message.

Domain 4: Quiz 3 Questions

1). After a training session to introduce a set of employees to a new process, you pass out an evaluation sheet to obtain feedback from the employees on the training session. Which of the following would be an inappropriate question?

A) Was the content accurate?
B) Did the instructor display enthusiasm?
C) Did the instructor maintain your interest?
D) Was the presentation organized/easy to follow?

2). Which of the following is not a reason to test?

A) To determine how well the worker can perform the objectives prior to training.
B) To be able to measure the learners' progress against other students.
C) To measure how well the student can perform the objectives during the training.
D) To determine how well the student can perform the objectives after training.

3). When you measure training program effectiveness, which of the following is the least valuable?

A) Behavior – what behaviors were changed as a result of the training
B) Knowledge – what skills were learned and demonstrated
C) Reaction – how the students liked the training
D) Interaction – how the students interacted and exchanged ideas in class

4). There are three main types of test that are administered during training. These are?

A) Multiple choice, essay and posttest
B) Multiple choice, essay and pretest
C) Pretest, review test and posttest
D) Multiple choice, essay and review test

5). Written documentation should be provided to each student who satisfactorily completes the training course. The documentation should include all the following except -
   A) Student's name.
   B) Student's Social Security Number
   C) Name and address of the training provider
   D) Statement that the student has successfully completed the course

6). The company has hired a new worker who was qualified as a powered truck operator at her previous company. What is the best method to determine the training needed for the operator?
   A) Enroll the operator in a formal school off site
   B) No training necessary, accept the other company's qualification
   C) Have the employee attend your company's initial training program.
   D) Verify the operator is competent with a performance evaluation.

7). When performing a training needs analysis, what is the fundamental question that a safety professional must ask?
   A) Will this organization's management commit to implementing this training?
   B) Will this organization's employees implement that which they learn during training?
   C) Will this organization accept the learning objectives?
   D) Will training resolve this organization's needs?

8). Which is an example of a well-constructed training objective?
   A) Students will understand the safety policy
   B) General industry training standards
   C) Each student can demonstrate the proper Energy Isolation Procedures
   D) Supervisors will be motivated deliver safety training

9). Which of the following is the least important outcome of safety and health training?
   A) Improved performance
   B) Fewer accidents
   C) Reduced costs
   D) Attitude adjustment

10). Which of the following training methods allows for the least amount of student-instructor interaction?
   A) Lecture
   B) Role playing
   C) Case study
   D) Facilitated discussion

11). One training technique especially useful when dealing with craft employees during safety and health training is the *case study*. Which of the following is the most correct concerning a case study?
   A) Case studies must always involve fictitious situations or accidents so that no one group or person will have hurt feelings
   B) Case studies should be written and passed out as handouts to be most effective
   C) Case studies are good problem solving tools
   D) Case studies involving real situations should only be used if they can be presented by the actual participants/victims

12). Adults learn best through:
   A) Seeing and listening.
   B) Saying.
   C) Seeing and doing.
   D) Listening and doing.

13). What are the two phases of effectively communicating risk to the public?
   A) Informing the public of the presence of the risk and involving the public in performing risk assessments.
   B) Identifying/locating the various loss scenarios for the public and educating the public on how the risk level was determined.
   C) Alerting/explaining a risk to the public and reassuring the public that the risk is being managed properly by describing what is being done to manage the risk.
   D) Disclosing the presence of a risk to the public and explaining to the public that the risk to the public is low.

14). Which major motivational condition best represents the characteristics and skills of a trainer providing effective feedback?
- A) Competence
- B) Inclusion
- C) Meaning
- D) Attitude

15). Reinforcement of desired behaviors is best accomplished by:
- A) Cash incentives
- B) Negative reinforcement at the end of the work shift
- C) Positive reinforcement as soon as possible
- D) Not required, adult's behaviors cannot be changed

16). Site Manager requests that CHST go to training to enhance skills related to safety on the job. The CHST should:
- A) Decline the training if possessing all necessary skills
- B) Attend first half of training to determine if relevant
- C) Go to training, as per BCSP Code of Ethics requiring continuous professional development
- D) Make verbal commitment, but do not attend training

17). When performing a training needs analysis, what is the fundamental question that a safety professional must ask?
- A) Will this organization's management commit to implementing this training?
- B) Will this organization's employees implement that which they learn during training?
- C) Will this organization accept the learning objectives?
- D) Will training resolve this organization's needs?

18). The most appropriate instructional method for improving interviewing skills, would be
- A) Lecture
- B) Demonstration
- C) Group discussion
- D) Role play

19). When developing a safety training program to train an operator on a specific piece of equipment, which is the least important?
   A) A description of how to use safety devices.
   B) How to identify equipment specific hazards
   C) A description of the design specifications for the equipment.
   D) When specific machine guarding can be removed.

20). Which of the following demonstrates a worker's knowledge of isolating a machine?
   A) Identifying the manufacturer of the machine
   B) Applying specific energy isolation locations and devices
   C) Reciting the company Lock out policy
   D) Locating the OSHA lock out standard

21). At minimum, documentation of training includes student name, topic outline, objectives, date and:
   A) Instructor name and qualifications
   B) Multi-media presentation
   C) Pre-and post test scores
   D) Literacy equivalency

22). Important minimum criteria for environmental, safety, and health trainers include:
   A) Documentation of relevant training and experience, compliance with regulatory requirements, and subject matter expertise.
   B) Accreditation, certification, and education.
   C) Subject matter expertise, training delivery skills, and continuing education.
   D) Knowledge, competence, and prior experience.

23). An Instructors actions taken to create an environment that supports and facilitates academic and social–emotional learning is called:
   A) Discipline management
   B) Classroom management
   C) Time management
   D) Program management

24). Small discussion groups are a useful adult training method and best described by which of the following statements?
   A) Easy for the instructor to control the quantity and type of information presented.
   B) Likely to encourage participation and stimulate interest.
   C) Very little risk of a dominant speaker controlling the discussion.
   D) Inappropriate for teaching creative problem-solving skills.

25). The most effective learning method for teaching chemical response technicians how to operate monitoring equipment is
   A) Demonstration.
   B) Lecture.
   C) Guided discussion.
   D) Self-directed.

Domain 4: Quiz 3 Answers

1). Answer A:

When presenting material that is new to a trainee, refrain from asking them to validate the content of the training program. Questions concerning the training environment, the instructor's skill and presentation are valid questions.

2). Answer B:

The three reasons to test are:
- to determine how well the students can perform the objectives prior to training.
- to measure how well the student can perform the objectives during the training.
- to determine how well the student can perform the objectives after training.

3). Answer C:

Reaction is the least valuable at the end of the training, since the student does not know the actual use of the skills or knowledge gained until they put it into action. That is why most training experts recommend a second critique after six months to obtain a valid reaction from the students.

4). Answer C:

The three main types of tests that are administered during a training session are the pretest, to determine baseline knowledge, review test, to determine progress and posttest to determine if the student has met the objectives.

5). Answer B:
Written documentation should be provided to each student who satisfactorily completes the training course. The documentation should include:
- Student's name.
- Course title.
- Course date.
- Statement that the student has successfully completed the course.
- Name and address of the training provider.
- An individual identification number for the certificate.

- List of the levels of personal protective equipment used by the student to complete the course.

This documentation may include a certificate and an appropriate wallet-sized laminated card with a photograph of the student and the above information. When such course certificate cards are used, the individual identification number for the training certificate should be shown on the card.

Recordkeeping. Training providers should maintain records listing the dates courses were presented, the names of the individual course attendees, the names of those students successfully completing each course, and the number of training certificates issued to each successful student. These records should be maintained for a minimum of five years after the date an individual participated in a training program offered by the training provider. These records should be available and provided upon the student's request or as mandated by law.

6). Answer D:

A performance evaluation is the best option to determine operator competency and provide hands on training in the work environment. CFR1910.178, Powered Industrial Trucks, requires anyone changing equipment or workplace location to meet the requirements outlined in the Refresher Training requirements (para 1910.178 (l)(4)). Only employees that are trained and authorized should operate industrial powered trucks.

7). Answer D:

According to *Developing Safety Training Programs,* the basic question is: Is this a training issue? The other questions are secondary.
Elements to Consider in Analyzing a Training Requirement

Element	Description
Statement of Training Need	The requester's statement of the training need.
Why is Training Required?	Identification of the requestor, the consequences of providing / not providing training, and the desired effects on the learners' job performance.
Who are the Learners?	Identification of the learners, their familiarity with the training content, and anticipated learner reactions to the training.
	The nature of the training content, possible

What's the Training Content?	resources, and anticipated difficulties in developing the content.
What are the Timing Issues?	The starting date, length / frequency of the training, and any known timing issues.
Where will the Training Be Conducted?	The location and number of learners, and an assessment of the space, equipment, and other resources that are needed and available.

When collecting data, focus on getting the necessary information for task analysis. This can be done by asking the right questions during data collection.

To Identify:	Ask the Question:
• Procedures, activities, steps.	What does the person do first? Next?
• Tools, materials.	What is used to perform the task?
• Operational systems	What is the task performed on?
• Cues	How do they know when to perform what?
• Work environment or conditions	Under what condition is the task performed?
• Performance standards	What is the standard of acceptable performance?

8). Answer C:

According to *Developing Safety Training Programs,* A learning objective must identify what the student will be able to do at the end of the training program. It is not part of the outline of the training program.

9). Answer D:

Training is primarily focused on behavior change. In education, the focus is on information about something that may or may not be used on the job. In training, the focus is also on how to do something properly and how to apply the new information and skills on the job. The primary benefits of safety and health training include:
- improved performance
- fewer incidents/accidents
- reduced costs

• reinforcement of the operational goals of the organization

Generally, attitude change is a secondary benefit to safety training. Exceptions may include human relations training using role play as an instructional strategy.

10). Answer A:

The benefits of the lecture is that you can impart information to a large group in a relative short time, however this leaves little time or opportunity for interaction between the trainee and the instructor.

Lecture Strategy			
Advantages	Limitations	Uses	Types of Objectives
Presents much information in a short time. Provides for instructor control. Good for introducing and summarizing new information. Can be entertaining.	Does not develop reasoning skills. Makes learners dependent on instructor. Is instructor-paced. Tends to be over-used. Can be boring.	Introduce new material. To summarize lesson. To establish instructor's expertise and leadership. Excellent for reflective observers. Enhanced by media.	Best for knowledge-level objectives, acquisition of facts.

11).   Answer C:

The case study is an especially effective technique for safety and health training, since it often illustrates the multi-causal aspects of accidents as well as the tragic consequences. The case study is an excellent problem solving technique. Normally case studies are presented to a group that has the goal of evaluating the mistakes made in the situation and providing real world solutions. The technique is particularly effective when the group is allowed to come to the conclusion that they can benefit from the mistakes of other construction contractors and thus prevent accidents. Real mishaps are effective case studies and should be used as often as possible to add credibility to the technique, but one must be aware of the sensitivities involved in tragic accidents.

Case Study			
Advantages	Limitations	Uses	Types of Objectives
Interactive Relevant Explore complex issues Applies new knowledge Can be entertaining.	Time consuming. May not see relevance	Develop analytic and problem solving skills Enhanced by pictures/media.	Best for knowledge-level objectives, Problem Solving

12)   Answer C:

The majority of adults learn best through seeing and doing. The Learning Pyramid illustrates information retention by activity.

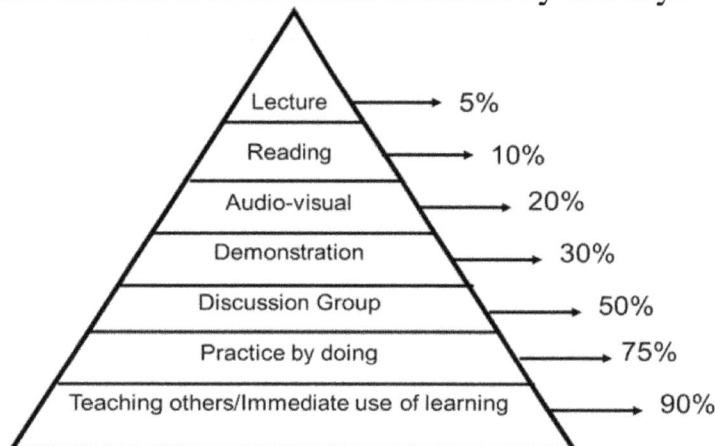

13)   Answer C:

Risk that affects the public must be explained to the public in a careful, planned way. First, the public must be alerted to the identity and magnitude of the risk in a straightforward, easy to understand way. Next, the public must be reassured that the risk is being managed and the steps that are being taken to manage the risk (in a straight forward, easy to understand way).

14)   Answer A:

The major motivational condition that best represents the characteristics and skills of a trainer providing effective feedback is Competence. Competency is generally defined in many resources as having the skills, knowledge and abilities to perform a task. A trainer must be competent in facilitation skills and subject matter to be able to provide effective learner feedback. ANSI/ASSE 490.1 **defines a Competent Training Professional as** a person prepared by education, training, or experience to develop and implement various elements of a training program. Also known in the standard as a Training Professional.

15)   Answer C:

There are two basic needs for reinforcement of desired behaviors. 1) provide positive reinforcement and; 2) the closer in time a reinforcement is associated with a behavior, the stronger the effect. Soon-Certain-Positive is the strongest motivator. To effect long term changes for minor infractions, punitive discipline is effective and appropriate. When discussing the "carrot and stick" management philosophy, contemporary literature suggest that the stick is no longer available, and the carrot is becoming less of an incentive.

16)   Answer C:

A safety professional should always look for opportunities to improve one's professional skill set as a life ling learner. The BCSP requires continuous professional development to maintain the CSHT by accumulating 20 continuing maintenance points per five-year cycle.

17)   Answer D:

According to *Developing Safety Training Programs,* the basic question is: Is this a training issue? The other questions are secondary. A determination shall be made as to whether training is the correct response to a given organizational need. In some cases, training will not fulfill the identified need. For example, a modified tool or workstation design rather than training may be needed to reduce potential for injuries.

18)   Answer D:

Role-playing refers to the changing of one's behavior to assume a role, either unconsciously to fill a social role, or consciously to act out an adopted role.

Training Method	Description	Advantages	Disadvantages
Case Study	Learners given hypothetical situation and asked to make a decision	Actively involves trainees, simulates reality, Can be observed	Precision needed, Can over-focus on content
Demonstration	Learners shown correct steps in completing a task	Aids understanding, Adds interest, Provides a model	Needs accuracy, Requires prep time
Guided/group Discussion	Trainer leads group in discussing a topic	Chance to share experiences, Can observe learning	Confusion, Domination by one or a few trainees
Lecture	Trainer orally presents new or review of old information	Keeps group together, Can be used with a large group, Can control time	Can be dull, Limited retention
Reading	Presents info in written format	Saves time, Consistency, Later use of "book"	Can be dull, pacing differences
Role-Play	In role-playing the learners act out a situation based on real life. Learners role-play the attitudes and behaviors involved in carrying out a task or job responsibility.	This method is especially useful when training is focused on how to work with people. Role-playing provides a more valid experience than merely talking about a problem.	The power of role playing is only harnessed when the role player receives EXPERT feedback Can create discomfort and anxiety. Less effective in large groups
Structured Exercises	Learners take part in exercises using new skills	Aids retention, Practices skills, Active involvement	Consumes class time, Requires prep time

19)   Answer C:

Design specifications are most likely overkill during a safety training session.. Teach them how to tell time, not how to build a watch.

20) Answer B:

Authorized workers must know the specific energy isolation locations and devices for each individual piece of equipment. Demonstrating the application of the isolation devices is the best performance measure. This should be part of initial training and the annual periodic review of the lock out program.

21) Answer A because

At minimum, documentation of training includes, student name, topic outline, objectives, date, instructor name and qualifications. Training records listing the dates courses were presented, the names of the individual course attendees, the names of those students successfully completing each course, and the number of training certificates issued to each successful student. Record retention policies may vary, but generally records should be maintained for a minimum of five years after the date of training. These records should be available and provided upon the student's request or as mandated by law.

22) Answer C:

EHS trainers should meet the minimum criteria as a subject matter expert, possess training delivery skills, and embrace continuing education.
Learning specialists must be able to develop learning objectives and select appropriate instructional methodologies that will foster increased knowledge, skills, and competencies and improve behaviors and attitudes on the part of the learners.
Characteristics of good trainers:

1.	Wants to be a trainer (wants to lead others).
2.	Relates well to others- a highly subjective criterion but essential, since working with people is what teaching is all about.
3.	Intelligence- must be able to quickly adapt and adjust to learners' answers and the context of the information being taught.
4.	Knows what he or she wants in a job- self-actualization rather than security and money.
5.	Willing to change self- changeable. Since change in others is the primary purpose of training, the learning specialist must be willing to demonstrate change or growth.
6.	Outgoing, enthusiastic, flair- the ability to make learning enjoyable and exiting.
7.	Analytical- if teaching from a manual, this is not necessary, but will be, if the learning specialist is asked to analyze who, what, and how he or she will teach.
8.	Self-awareness- this criterion relates to criterion V because it reveals a person's self-knowledge. Awareness is essential, because being aware of anything is the first step in the change process.

9. Secure within self- being satisfied with oneself is important because it demonstrates internal congruence, an attribute needed in more managers, supervisors, and employees.

10. Experience- not in teaching, which is expected of all learning specialist, but in the subject matter they are teaching.

23) Answer B:

Classroom management as the actions taken to create an environment that supports and facilitates academic and social–emotional learning. Instructors must (1) develop caring, supportive relationships with and among students; (2) organize and implement instruction in ways that optimize students' access to learning; (3) use group management methods that encourage students' engagement in academic tasks; (4) promote the development of students' social skills and self–regulation; and (5) use appropriate interventions to assist students with behavior problems. Another source describes classroom management as a process consisting of key tasks that instructors must attend to in order to develop an environment conducive to learning. These tasks include: (1) organizing the physical environment, (2) establishing rules and routines, (3) developing caring relationships, (4) implementing engaging instruction and (5) preventing and responding to discipline problems

24) Answer B:

A discussion is usually effective in engaging learners and encouraging participation. Peer learning is one of the most direct benefits resulting from the discussion method. Discussions can involve small groups (2-8 participants) or structured for larger groups. Typically discussions center around problems, questions, ideas or issues presented to the group for consideration and verbal exploration.

25) Answer A:

A trainer begins the demonstration method with performing an activity or a behavior while learners observe and then later perform. Demonstrations are useful tools to provide learners with the opportunity to observe prior to practicing critical hands on skills.

Domain 4: Quiz 4 Questions

1). Which of the following is the most important consideration for determining a delivery method?

A) Guarantee the relevance of training goals.

B) Appropriate to the target audience and training objectives.

C) Establish criteria for completion in the course description.

D) Identify the student-instructor ratio and training materials.

2). What is the best source for instructing employees in how to operate a tool safely?

A) OSHA

B) The Supervisor

C) The manufacturer instruction manual

D) The site safety officer

3). During a lecture presentation, the LCD projector will not operate. In the absence of power point, what should you do?

A) Reach into your trainer's toolbox and use other methods to convey the information.

B) Cancel or post pone the class and get a projector.

C) Proclaim your dissatisfaction with the facilities and equipment to the class.

D) Have the participants read the class handout notes.

4). Why should supervisors discuss the results of safety inspections with their employees?

A) To give positive reinforcement for good work practice and discuss hazards and corrective measures.

B) Determine disciplinary actions

C) To find the root cause.

D) To report accidents and near misses.

5). It is a generally accepted theory in accident prevention that the attitude of supervisors and managers can affect the actions of foreman and employees. Which of the following best describes that relationship?

A) Supervisor's attitudes have no effect on employees.

B) Supervisor's attitudes have little effect on employees.

C) Supervisor's attitude has a direct influence on employees.

D) Supervisor's attitudes have a direct influence, which cannot be changed

6). The plaintiff's attorney contacts a CHST with specific subject matter expert witness for a highly publicized court case. The attorney offers to compensate the CHST with 5% of the settlement if the plaintiff's case is successful. The **most** ethical action is to:

    A) Accept the offer with an additional upfront retainer fee.
    B) Reject the offer and report the attorney to the BCSP.
    C) Counter the offer with an hourly fee schedule.
    D) Counter the offer requesting 10% of the settlement.

7). Once you obtained your CHST, you must maintain your currency in the safety and health arena. This is monitored by the BCSP by the Continuance of Certification program. All the following are ways to obtain certification points except:

    A) Engaged in acceptable, professional safety practice for at least 25% of a 40 hour work week
    B) Serving as an officer on approved technical/professional committees or safety organizations
    C) Contributions to the safety body of knowledge through publications, presentations and patents
    D) Drafting CHST examination questions at workshops or by submitting them individually

8). Once you obtained your CHST, you must maintain your currency in the safety and health arena. This is monitored by the BCSP by the Certification Maintenance program. If you fail to meet your required 20 points in five years you must:

    A) Obtain 50 points in the next five year period
    B) Complete 20 college credits to be reinstated
    C) Retake the CHST exam
    D) Resubmit an application for reevaluation

9). As a CHST, you are working as a consultant for a company and identify a condition that poses serious risk to the employees. You notify the client of serious safety concerns and he tells you that he does not have the money to fix the condition. The most ethical response to this situation is to:

    A) Report the situation to OSHA.
    B) Keep good documentation of this situation.
    C) Discuss the situation with the client to find a solution.
    D) You have informed the client and your responsibility has ended.

10). The National Society of Professional Engineers publishes a set of fundamental canons that is expects its members to follow. These have been copied by many safety organizations as their standards. They include all the following except:
   A) Hold paramount the safety, health and welfare of the public.
   B) Avoid deceptive acts.
   C) Perform services in any safety area requested.
   D) Act for each employer or client as faithful agents or trustees.

11). If CHSTs were petitioning to the state to have only certified individual recognized as safety and health professionals, this would be an example of
   A) Title Protection.
   B) Professional Registration.
   C) A Title Act.
   D) Professional Competence Standard.

12). You are conducting a safety inspection of a manufacturing plant in the southwest and mentoring a graduate safety professional(GSP) intern. During the inspection an employee is observed, without eye protection, working at a bench installing parts. This is not a hazardous operation, but it is a posted "eye protection" area. Which of the following is the **best** course of action?
   A) Contact the supervisor and discuss the situation.
   B) Test the graduate safety professional skills to handle the situation.
   C) Confront the employee and determine "Why" eye protection is not being used.
   D) Send an email to notify the CEO and the supervisor.

13). When the primary contracting party assumes all liability and holds harmless the 2nd party is the definition of :
   A) Errors and omissions
   B) Res ipsa loquitur
   C) Indemnity
   D) Contract clause

14). Charges of unethical conduct against a CHST must be:
   A) Presented in front of the entire board
   B) Be submitted on an approved form available from the board
   C) Be submitted within a year of the alleged offense
   D) Be written and notarized

15). A worker has returned to work after an injury with a "light work" letter from his doctor. The supervisor told the worker that he would have to do his normal job and ignore the doctor's orders. Your first action should be:

    A) Report the supervisor to the CEO
    B) Discuss the situation with the SH&E Director
    C) Discuss the situation with the supervisor
    D) Tell the employee to disregard the supervisors orders

16). Insurance contracts are unilateral, meaning that only the insurer makes legally enforceable promises in the contract. The insured is not required to pay premiums, but the insurer is required to pay benefits under contract if the insured has paid the premiums and met certain other basic provisions. Which terms represent the general parts of an insurance contract?

    A) Declarations, Definitions, Insuring agreement, Exclusions, Conditions, Endorsements.
    B) Incontestability, Definitions, Conditions, Declarations.
    C) Investigation, Exclusions, Conditions, Privity.
    D) Endorsements, Definitions, Executor, Declaration.

17). A site superintendent requests that the CHST conduct samples on the dust from a grinding operation. The CHST has no experience with collecting samples. The CHST should:

    A) Notify superintendent that CHST is not qualified and recommend the company gets a qualified person to collect samples
    B) Read up on specific materials and perform sampling
    C) Recommend proceeding with job without sampling
    D) Put crew in respirators

18). A CHST must accept responsibility for their continued professional development by acquiring and maintaining competence through continuing education, experience, professional training, and:

    A) Monitoring safety websites.
    B) Maintaining a presence on social networks.
    C) Keeping current on relevant legal issues.
    D) Keeping a regular Internet blog.

19). Which of the following best describes an expectation of the CHST Code of Ethics?

    A) Perform their supervisory roles in a manner to protect their employer.

    B) Perform their safety roles using their knowledge and skills to further the safety of employees, employers, the public and the environment.

    C) Avoiding circumstances that might compromise their employer or their employees.

    D) Maintaining confidentiality of all information that might impugn their employer or client.

20). An agreement or contract in which one party agrees to hold the other free from the responsibility for any liability or damage that might arise out of the transaction involved is called a:

    A) Strict liability

    B) Hold harmless agreement

    C) Negligence

    D) Exclusive remedy

21). A food processing plant has a storm water containment pond that is not fenced. If a child drowns in the pond, what is the legal doctrine a plaintiff could use in a lawsuit?

    A) Attractive nuisance

    B) Res ipsa loquitur

    C) Obvious peril

    D) Foreseeability

22). Employee unions can impact safety:

    A) Negatively when there is insistence for engineering control as a substitute for disciplinary action.

    B) Negatively when union leaders have a role in safety training.

    C) Positively when employees bargain for safety incentive programs based upon reducing accident rates.

    D) Positively when workers have more direct involvement in reducing workplace hazards.

23). The "Fellow Servant Rule" involved which of the following principles:
- A) Employer must establish a "two-man" rule
- B) Employees were not responsible for each other
- C) Rules were established for more than one worker
- D) Employer was not responsible for injuries caused by another worker

24). A guest at a theme park is injured when sliding down a water slide. Which best describes the legal defense in a tort lawsuit?
- A) Assumption of risk
- B) Caveat emptor
- C) Express liability
- D) Negligence

25). Management has increased work hours and is pushing for more productivity. As CHST, you are concerned about some of the safety risks associated with this production schedule. You should:
- A) Report concern to the US Department of Labor (DOL)
- B) Tell workers to launch a work slow down
- C) Inform/communicate increased hazards due to increased production and verify that risk is acceptable
- D) Do not challenge the management; accept the production schedule

Domain 4: Quiz 4 Answers

1) Answer B:

Multiple delivery methods may be used in a single training course or event and all of the answer choices are valid considerations. The most important is to ensure that the delivery method is appropriate for the audience and accomplishes the training objectives.

2) Answer C:

Manufacturer's recommendations are the primary resource for operating tools and equipment. Training programs should incorporate the manufactures operating manual. Supervisors may be in the best position to deliver the training, but they should not be expected to be instructional designers.

3) Answer A:

To be an effective trainer/facilitator, one must have a go-to toolkit. While multi-media presentations are great tools, death by power point is the result of this technology being overused as a crutch for poor facilitation skills. Some of the best presentations delivered by skilled facilitators have been out of spontaneity due to technical difficulties. On the other hand, such disruption can be disastrous for a one dimensional, inflexible, or novice instructor. Bottom line: Have a backup plan.

4) Answer A:

Supervisors should continuously give positive reinforcement for good work practice and discuss hazards and corrective measures.

5) Answer C:

Supervisor's attitude has a direct influence on the employee's safety performance.

6) Answer C:

You must avoid the appearance of a "conflict of interest" to maintain your credibility. A flat fee schedule demonstrates that you have no stake in the case outcome. Conduct your professional relations by the highest standards of integrity and avoid compromise of their professional judgment by conflicts of interest.

7). Answer A:

CM point rules are outlined in the Certification Maintenance Guide and include the following categories:

      i. Safety and Health Practice (35% of 30 hour week)
      ii. Health & Safety Organization Membership
      iii. Technical/Professional Committee Service, Safety & Health Organizations Offices
      iv. Professional Publications, Papers, Technical Presentations and Patent
      v. Preparation of Examination Questions
      vi. Professional Development Conferences
      vii. Continuing Education Courses
      viii. College or University Courses
      ix. Academic Degrees
      x. Re-examination

8). Answer C:

CM rules are outlined in the Certification Maintenance Guide and it states:

"A failure to meet your CM requirements results in your OHST or CHST certification being revoked. You may re-acquire the certification by paying the examination fee (reapplication is not required) and passing the current OHST or CHST examination. You must complete this activity within five years of being notified that the certification is no longer valid.

If more than five years passes after losing your OHST or CHST certification because CM requirements were not met, you must seek the certification as a new applicant."

9). Answer C:

Professional responsibility is to advise the client of the risks of serious injuries and help the client to find a solution.

10). Answer C:

According to the National Society of Professional Engineers Fundamental Canons, engineers, in the fulfillment of their professional duties, shall:

- Hold paramount the safety, health and welfare of the public.
- Perform services only in areas of their competence.
- Issue public statements only in an objective and truthful manner.
- Act for each employer or client as faithful agents or trustees.
- Avoid deceptive acts.
- Conduct themselves honorably, responsibly, ethically, and lawfully so as to enhance the honor, reputation, and usefulness of the profession.

By maintaining these canons, it assures the public and others that you have achieved these professional standards.

11). Answer A:

A Title Act is the method a state would choose to enact specific Title Protection. The purpose of title protection according to an ASSE Position Statement is to "provide legal recognition to the profession of safety as well as provide assurance to the public that individuals representing themselves as being involved in the profession of safety **as safety professionals,** have met the listed minimum qualifications, thereby protecting the public health and safety from harm." If an individual uses the CHST designation without first being certified by the BCSP, that individual may be barred from pursuing any BCSP certification and/or be sued.

12). Answer A:

The first action is to protect the worker. Stopping the operation and discussing with the worker is most appropriate in imminent danger situations. In this case, you should be to contact the supervisor who has control of the workplace and discuss the hazards of the job and PPE requirements. Additionally, mentor demonstrated leadership by involving key shareholders and decision makers.

13). Answer C:

To explain an indemnity agreement, it is first necessary to define the term "indemnity." Indemnity is defined as "a duty to make good any loss, damage, or liability incurred by another. Indemnity has the general meaning of "hold harmless;" that is, one party holds the other harmless for some loss or damage. There are some variations of meaning for the term "indemnity". An indemnity agreement (sometimes called a "hold harmless agreement" can be a contract or a section of a contract. In these cases, an indemnity agreement is contract language that indemnifies (holds harmless) one of the parties in a contract for specific actions that might cause damage to the other party.

14).   Answer D:

Complaints should be submitted as soon as possible and must be written describing the behavior or circumstances and be notarized. The first step the board will take will be to verify that the complaint is valid.

15).   Answer C:

Your basic job is as an advisor to the management structure and the workforce, therefore the first action should be to discuss the situation with the supervisor and see if he will reconsider. Remember that before you do anything that is out of your scope of authority, you should always consult your supervisor.

16).   Answer A:

The parts of an insurance contract include:
- Declarations - identify who is an insured, insured's address, insuring company, what risks or property are covered, policy limits (amount of insurance), any applicable deductibles, policy period and premium amount. These are usually provided on a form that is completed by the insurer based on the insured's application and attached on top of or inserted within the first few pages of a standard policy form.
- Definitions - define important terms used in policy language.
- Insuring agreement - describes the covered perils, or risks assumed, or nature of coverage, or makes some reference to the contractual agreement between insurer and insured. It summarizes the major promises of the insurance company, as well as stating what is covered.
- Exclusions – negates coverage from Insuring Agreement by describing property, perils, hazards or losses arising from specific causes which are **not** covered by the policy.
- Conditions - provisions, rules of conduct, duties and obligations required for

coverage. If policy conditions are not met, the insurer can deny the claim.

- Endorsements - additional forms attached to the policy form that modify it in some way, either unconditionally or upon existence of some condition. Endorsements can make policies difficult to read for nonlawyers; they may modify or delete clauses located several pages earlier in the standard insuring agreement, or even modify each other. Because it is very risky to allow nonlawyer underwriters to directly rewrite core policy language with word processors. Insurers usually direct underwriters to modify standard forms by attaching endorsements preapproved by counsel for various common modifications.

17). Answer A:

The CHST code of ethics states that a CHST should perform safety responsibilities and assignments **only** in areas of their competence.

18). Answer C:

An CHST should always look for opportunities to improve one's professional skill set. According to the BCSP Code of Ethics, a CSP should accept responsibility for their continued professional development by acquiring and maintaining competence through continuing education, experience, professional training and keeping current on relevant legal issues.

19). Answer B:

"Perform their safety roles using their knowledge and skills to further the safety of employees, employers, the public and the environment" best describes an expectation of the CHST Code of Ethics

20). Answer B:

A *Hold Harmless (Indemnity) Agreement* is used between two parties to establish that the indemnitee is protected from any unforeseen liabilities, losses, claims or damages during their involvement in an activity. A Hold Harmless Agreement is developed to prevent law suits by assigning liability in a contract. Hold harmless means that if there is a problem and a suit later, one party shields or "holds harmless" the other. A hold harmless clause is a statement in a legal contract stating that an individual or organization is not liable for any injuries or damages caused to the individual signing the contract.

An individual may be asked to sign a hold harmless agreement when undertaking an activity that involves risk for which the enabling entity does not want to be legally or financially responsible.

Strict liability is the concept whereby the plaintiff need not show negligence or fault to prove liability.

Negligence is the failure to exercise a reasonable amount of care or to carry out a legal duty so that injury or property damage occurs to another. An example would be you were a landlord and did not provide adequate security and the renter was robbed.

Exclusive Remedy: State workers' compensation statutes gave employees a definite remedy for injuries and diseases arising out of or suffered in the course of their employment. In exchange for a definite recovery, the workers' compensation remedy is exclusive, that is, with just a few exceptions, a worker's right of recovery against the employer is limited to the benefits provided by the workers' compensation law. The employee may not sue in tort.

21).   Answer A:

The **attractive nuisance** doctrine applies to the law of torts, in the United States. It states that a landowner may be held liable for injuries to children trespassing on the land if the injury is caused by an object on the land that is likely to attract children **Tort** is a wrongful act or a failure to exercise due care that results in damage or injury in the broadest sense.

A manufacturer or distributor would not have to label a large blade hunting knife because the product involves an **obvious peril**, sometimes called an obvious hazard that is well known to the public.

22).   Answer D:

Unions are important participants in a safety culture. They want to eliminate injuries that harm their members. To do that, unions favor changes to the workplace that make it safer. Unions have challenged the reliance of some employers upon the discipline of individual workers for safety-related behaviors. Unions assert that the disciplining of individuals for errors is far less effective than a program of pre-incident planning, risk assessment, and engineering controls. A fail-safe device or design makes the errors less likely to cause injuries. The desirable investment in workplace design change that the union prefers would render the machine quieter, the floor safer, and the equipment guards impregnable to removal or evasion. This emphasis shifts the issues away from discipline of errant people to the needs for engineers to devise built-in constraints on peoples' capacity for accepting risk or making foolish judgments. Unions' effectiveness in collective bargaining for safety issues varies with economic situations, and with the urgency felt by an individual local bargaining team to assert safety issues. *If the union is able to win concessions on safety issues, the enhanced union-management effort probably increases the likelihood that workers will support the culture and act with greater awareness of safety.* If work teams are used, the training of work teams for safety should include the support of union leadership such as the local president or shop steward for the safety program.

23)   Answer D:

The Fellow Servant Rule was a defense which, prior to the enactment of workers compensation laws, could be used by an employer to protect his self when sued by an employee for damages on account of injury caused by one or more fellow employees.

24)   Answer A:

Assumption of risk is a defense in the law of torts, which bars or reduces a plaintiff's right to recovery against a negligent tortfeasor if the defendant can demonstrate that the plaintiff voluntarily and knowingly assumed the risks at issue inherent to the dangerous activity in which he was participating at the time of his or her injury. What is usually meant by assumption of risk is more precisely termed *primary* or "express" assumption of risk. It occurs when the plaintiff has either expressly or implicitly relieved the defendant of the duty to mitigate or relieve the risk causing the injury from which the cause of action arises. It operates as a complete bar to liability on the theory that upon assumption of the risk, there is no longer a duty of care running from the defendant to the plaintiff; without a duty owed by the defendant, there can be no negligence on his part. However, primary assumption of risk is not a blanket exemption from liability for the operators of a dangerous activity. The *specific* risk causing the injury must have been known to, and appreciated by, the plaintiff in order for primary assumption of risk to apply. Also, assumption of risk does not absolve a defendant of liability for reckless conduct.

Negligence is the failure to exercise a reasonable amount of care or to carry out a legal duty so that injury or property damage occurs to another.

Caveat Emptor. [Let the buyer beware.] A warning that notifies a buyer that the goods he or she is buying are "as is," or subject to all defects.

Breach of warranty-based product liability claims usually focus on one of three types: (1) breach of an express warranty, (2) breach of an implied warranty of merchantability, and (3) breach of an implied warranty of fitness for a particular purpose. **Express warranty** claims focus on express statements by the manufacturer or the seller concerning the product (e.g., "This chainsaw is useful to cut turkeys").

25)   Answer C:

Informing/communicating to upper management the increased hazards due to increased production and verifying that risk is acceptable is the best solution.

Domain 4: Quiz 5 Questions

1). Professional ethics refers to:
   A) A set of principles and standards that guide the actions of professionals that are often referenced in civil or criminal cases involving professional conduct.
   B) The laws that the professional must comply with or face possible civil and criminal charges.
   C) A set of bylaws established to assure the members of an organization must follow.
   D) Voluntary rules expected of members of professional associations.

2). You are the supervisor at the site of a 15-foot underground pipe installation. The final connections have been made, all workers and shoring have been removed. If the project is completed by today's deadline your company will receive an on time bonus. A subcontractor notifies you that he has left an expensive laser pipe level in the trench. Which of the following is the best course of action?
   A) Refuse to put anybody else at risk and enter the hole yourself to retrieve the equipment.
   B) Direct the equipment operator use the backhoe and retrieve the subcontractor's equipment.
   C) Direct the equipment operator to fill the trench as the subcontractor's tools are not your problem.
   D) Inform the subcontractor that your crew will take a 10-minute break so he can enter the trench.

3). Which of the following identifies the four mandatory elements for any legal contract?
   A) Consent, legal tender, parties, consideration.
   B) Management, labor, money, contract.
   C) Agreement, consideration, purpose, legal tender.
   D) Agreement, consideration, purpose, competent parties.

4). A CSP and licensed professional engineer asks a supervisor to informally review a series of fall protection plans for a warehouse construction project. The supervisor has adequately reviewed these types of plans for years, although without an engineering degree or formal fall protection system design education. Which statement most represents a reasonable interpretation of the BCSP Code of Ethics?
- A) A CHST is qualified by exam to and permitted to approve employer safety programs.
- B) A CHST is permitted to participate in a review of any construction related activity.
- C) The BCSP Code of Ethics permits only licensed professional engineers to determine whether other safety professionals have qualifications for reviewing their work.
- D) The BCSP Code of Ethics permits CHSTs to engage in work when they are qualified by experience in the specific technical fields involved, as well as by education.

5). Site Superintendent asks a CHST to evaluate the injury records for a 1 Million-Man-Hours-With-No-Lost-Time Accident Award. Upon review, the CHST discovers that a case involving 3 days away from work was not categorized correctly. The CHST should:
- A) Report the misclassification to the site superintendent.
- B) Allow recognition to continue.
- C) Notify the federal authorities.
- D) Do not issue the award.

6). A CHST notices hazardous behavior on the job site, he/she should
- A) Communicate the observation at the appropriate level.
- B) Confront the offenders.
- C) Send an email to the crew.
- D) Document the observation submit a report to human resources.

7). Lecture would be the most efficient means for:
- A) Putting out technical information like regulatory changes
- B) Teaching inter-personal skills
- C) Exploring group dynamics
- D) Getting a group of people to bond

8). What is the most effective coaching method
   A) Group
   B) Individual
   C) Feedback
   D) Disciplinary

9). Who would primarily have a coaching and feedback role after training?
   A) Safety director
   B) Supervisor
   C) Fellow worker
   D) Subcontractor

10). You are a CHST and you notice that hearing protection use is down, what should you do?
   A) Ask employees about fit & comfort
   B) Ask employees their opinion of PPE
   C) Review injury log
   D) Discipline employees

11). What is the minimum training a new employee must have for safety orientation?
   A) PPE training
   B) Confined space entry training
   C) First aid / first responder training
   D) Specific hazards of job and how to protect self

12). When are employees required to receive HAZCOM training?
   A) Initially and before working with new chemical
   B) Monthly
   C) Annually
   D) Semi-Annually

13). When is an employer required to provide First Aid / CPR training?
   A) They are never required to provide this training
   B) After a major event in case of another
   C) Anytime they have a fire brigade
   D) When medical care not readily accessible

14). What is the supervisor's primary role in training?
   A) Train the trainer
   B) Coaching and feedback
   C) Evaluation and enforcement
   D) Designer and facilitator

15). Safety training is best implemented by:
   A) The CHST because they are the most knowledgeable
   B) The job Foreman because he has the most authority
   C) The OHSA inspector they are the experts
   D) The Supervisor integrating it into all other training

16). What is the best way to convince others to accept a potential improvement?
   A) Tell them it is required
   B) Try to tie it to a regulatory requirement
   C) Demonstrate how the intervention will reduce costs or save money
   D) Try use a moral or character argument

17). If a training session is 30% lecture and 70 % hands on, it is considered:
   A) Application based
   B) Exercise based
   C) Learning based
   D) Interactive based

18). What would be the best method for evaluating an employee's recall of facts?
   A) True or false question test
   B) Multiple choice question test
   C) Matching answer test
   D) Short essay answer test

19). As a CHST, how many re-certification points will you need to earn?
   A) 20 over 5 years
   B) 20 annually
   C) 5 points a year
   D) 50 over 5 years

20). A worker is observed staring off into space while operating equipment is **most** likely:

   A) Bored.
   B) Complacent.
   C) Untrained.
   D) Ignorant.

Domain 4: Quiz 5 Answers

1)   Answer A:

Ethics refers to a set of principles and standards that guide the actions of professionals that are often referenced in civil or criminal cases involving professional conduct. A basic definition of ethics is: moral principles or practice. Professional ethics require consideration of additional areas including, professional values, culture, acceptable standards of behavior and legality. Professionals will likely face ethical dilemmas during their career. Some day-to-day ethical dilemmas are simple to determine the correct course of action; others are not as clear.

2)   Answer B:

The best resolution is to have the backhoe operator retrieve equipment. Entering an unprotected 15-foot-deep excavation is clear violation of the regulations and allowing the contractor to enter an unprotected trench is unethical. If an option is legal then another good measure is to determine if it is balanced. The decision to tell the subcontractor, "tough - it is your own fault," is not clearly balanced. A skilled backhoe operator will likely be able to retrieve the equipment without damaging it and complete the project on time.

3)   Answer D:

A legal contract must have four parts:
- Agreement
- Consideration
- Purpose
- Competent parties

4)   Answer D:

The standard in the BCSP Code of Ethics states that a CHST shall "Perform safety responsibilities and assignments only in areas of their competence." Competence can be achieved through formal training, on-the-job training and experience.

5)   Answer A:

The best solution in this example is to communicate the discrepancy with the site superintendent.

6)   Answer A:

Hazardous behavior being noticed by anyone should be immediately addressed—especially by safety people. HOW you address it could be the key to preventing its recurrence. "Confronting" people about behavior seldom results in them changing that behavior. Likewise, reporting it to others seldom results positively because it is often viewed as a 'snitch' or 'tattle-tell'. Ignoring the behavior will just reinforce it as acceptable. The best approach is to ask the person about what they did and if they noticed the potential hazard. Asking their opinion and insight will initiate a non-confrontational conversation in which you might be able to convince them there is a better way.

7)   Answer A:

Lecture is the most efficient means listed as options for communicating a lot of technical information to a large group.

8)   Answer C:

Studies have shown that immediate and positive feedback is the most effective way of getting people to change their behavior.

9)   Answer B:

Supervisors are always the primary coach in the workplace. Highly effective organizations are those where supervisors are effective at providing targeted feedback.

10)   Answer B:

We chose to "ask the employees their opinion". While asking employees about fit and comfort is not a bad idea—either of those might be the reason they are not using the PPE, that question will not illicit as much information from them as asking a more open-ended question. If the fit and comfort was not an issue to them, they might not offer what is an issue. Asking their opinion should lead them directly to the issue that each employee feels is important.

11)   Answer D:

With so little information, this is a difficult question to answer. However, in every employment situation the employer is at risk of a citation—if nothing else from the general duty clause—if they do not train their employees on known hazards and how those are to be mitigated.

12)   Answer A:

OSHA does not require employers to provide HAZCOM training annually, semi-annually or monthly. It is required prior to an employee is exposed to chemicals in the workplace and when a new chemical is brought into the workplace.

13)   Answer D:

29 CFR 1926.50(c) states: "In the absence of an infirmary clinic, hospital, or physician, that is reasonably accessible in terms of time and distance to the worksite, which is available for the treatment of injured employees, a person who has a valid certificate in first-aid training from the U.S. Bureau of Mines, the American Red Cross, or equivalent training that can be verified by documentary evidence, shall be available at the worksite to render first aid."

14)   Answer B:

While supervisors are often trainers themselves, their primary role is as a coach or mentor providing feedback and constant guidance or reinforcement of the topics covered in training. They often unofficially evaluate the effectiveness of training by observing worker behavior and enforce the concepts through accountability. They are seldom designers or facilitators of training and rarely train others to be trainers.

15)   Answer D:

It is always recommended to integrate Safety topics into the normal operational management process. Of the options given here, integrating safety into the operational training is ideal.

16)   Answer C:

All the options offered here are viable; however, the **best** way to get others to accept it is to tie it to a monetary benefit.

17) Answer D:

Interactive training is training that follows the 70/30 rule where 70% is some sort of hands-on where the learning is applying the concepts that they just learned from lecture, which is limited to 30% of the total time.

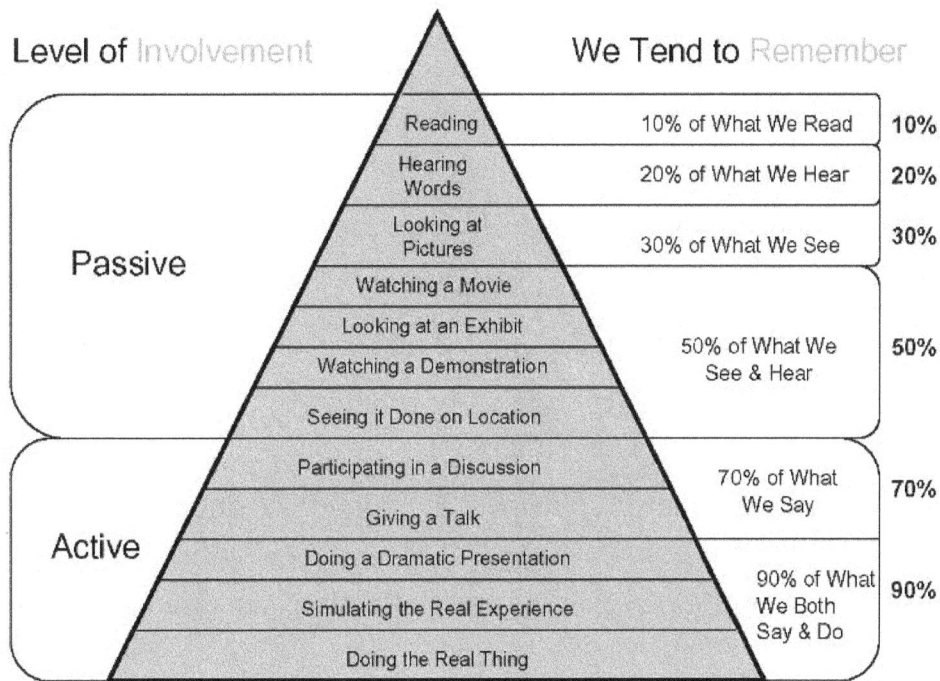

Based on the work of Edgar Dale and Robert Felder

18) Answer B:

While both true/false and multiple-choice questions are suitable for testing recall, true/false questions are less reliable than multiple choice. Essay questions are not suited for recall.

19) Answer A:

BCSP requires 20 recertification points for CHSTs to retain their designation. These are required to be submitted every 5 years.

20) Answer B:

An employee staring off into space is obviously distracted by something. S/he may be bored but must be complacent to the potential hazards of the area to allow themselves to become so distracted.

References

These published references provide reasonable coverage on the subject matter associated with the CHST4 Examination Blueprint. Examination items are not necessarily taken directly from these sources. You may have alternate editions of these references in your library that also present acceptable coverage on the subject matter, as well as other useful references.

Elements of Ergonomics Programs: A Primer Based on Workplace Evaluations of Musculoskeletal Disorders

Cohen, A. L., Gjessing, C.C., et al. (1997). Diane Publishing Co.; Darby, PA.

14 Elements of a Successful Safety & Health Program

National Safety Council. (1994). National Safety Council; Washington, D.C.

Accident Investigation Techniques; 2nd Edition

Oakley, J. S. & American Society of Safety Engineers. (2012). American Society of Safety Engineers; Des Plaines, IL.

Accident Prevention Manual for Business & Industry: Administration & Programs; 14th Edition

Hagan, P.E., J. F., Montgomery, et al. (2015). National Safety Council; Itasca, IL.

Accident Prevention Manual for Business & Industry: Engineering and Technology

Hagan, P.E., J. F., Montgomery, et al. (2012). National Safety Council; Itasca, IL.

Accident Prevention Manual for Business & Industry: Security Management

Lack, R. W. (1997). National Safety Council; Itasca, IL.

Advanced Safety Management: Focusing on Z10 & Serious Injury Prevention

Manuele, F. A. (2008). John Wiley & Sons, Inc.; Hoboken, NJ.

Analyzing Safety System Effectiveness; 3rd Edition

Petersen, D. (1996). Van Nostrand Reinhold; New York, NY.

BCSP Code of Ethics

Board of Certified Safety Professionals. (2013). Retrieved from http://www.bcsp.org/Portals/0/Assets/DocumentLibrary/BCSPcodeofethics.pdf.

BCSP Recertification Guide

Board of Certified Safety Professionals. (2018). Recertification Guide. Retrieved from http://www.bcsp.org/Portals/0/Assets/DocumentLibrary/RecertGuide.pdf.

Chemical Protective Clothing; 2nd Edition

Anna, D. H. (2003). American Industrial Hygiene Association Press; Fairfax, VA.

Complete Confined Spaces Handbook

Rekus, J. (1994). CRC Press; Boca Raton, FL.

Complete Guide to Training Delivery, The: A Competency-Based Approach

King, S. B., Rothwell, W. J., et al. (2001). AMACOM; New York, NY.

Construction Safety Management and Engineering; 2nd Edition

Hill, D. C. (2014). American Society Safety Engineers; Des Plaines, IL.

Construction Safety Planning

MacCollum, D. (1995). John Wiley & Sons, Inc.; Hoboken, NJ.

Contractor Safety Management

Smith, G. W. (2013). CRC Press; Boca Raton, FL.

Definitions, Conversions, and Calculations for Occupational Safety and Health Professionals; 3rd Edition

Finucane, E. W. (2006). CRC Press; Boca Raton, FL.

Developing an Effective Safety Culture: A Leadership Approach

Roughton, J. E. & Mercurio, J. J. (2002). Butterworth-Heinemann; Boston, MA.

Emergency Incident Management Systems: Fundamentals and Applications

Molino, L. N. (2006). John Wiley & Sons, Inc.; Hoboken, NJ.

Encyclopedia of Occupational Safety and Health, The

Stellman, J. (1998). International Labor Office; Geneva, Switzerland.

Excavation Systems: Planning, Design, & Safety

Turner, J. M. (2009). McGraw-Hill; New York, NY.

Fall Protection & Scaffolding Safety

Drennan, G. (2000). Government Institutes, Scarecrow Press; Lanham, MD.

Fire Protection Handbook: Volume I & II; 20th Edition

Cote, A. E., Hall, J. R., et al. (2008). National Fire Protection Association; Quincy, MA.

Fire Safety Management Handbook; 3rd Edition

Della-Giustina, D. (2014). CRC Press; Boca Raton, FL.

Fitting the Task to the Human: A Textbook of Occupational Ergonomics; 5th Edition

Kroemer, K.H.E. & E. Grandjean (1997). CRC Press; Boca Raton, FL.

Fundamentals of Fire Protection for the Safety Professional

Ferguson, L. H. & Janicak, C. A. (2005). Government Institutes; Lanham, MD.

Fundamentals of Industrial Hygiene; 6th Edition

Plog, B. A. & Quinlan, P. (2012). National Safety Council; Itasca, IL.

Globally Harmonized System of Classification and Labeling of Chemicals; 5th Revised Edition

United Nations. (2013). United Nations; New York, NY.

Guides for Managing Crystalline Silica Control Programs in Construction

Zuckerman, N., Wanzer, K., et al. (2004). Retrieved from https://www.silica-safe.org/training-and-other-resources/manuals-and-guides/asset/2-Training-Guides-for-Manag- ing-Crystalline-Silica-Control-Programs-in-Construction.pdf

Handbook of Occupational Safety & Health; 2nd Edition

DiBerardinis, L. J. (1999). John Wiley & Sons, Inc.; New York, NY.

Handbook of Rigging: Lifting, Hoisting, and Scaffolding for Construction and Industrial Operations; 5th Edition

MacDonald, J. A., Rossnagel, W. E., et al. (2009). McGraw Hill; New York, NY.

Handbook of Safety & Health for the Service Industry: Industrial Safety & Health for Infrastructure Services

Reese, C.D. (2008). CRC Press; Boca Raton, FL.

Hazardous Materials Management Desk Reference

Cox, Doye B. (2000). McGraw-Hill; New York, NY.

Human Safety and Risk Management: A Psychological Perspective; 3rd Edition

Glendon, A. I. & Clarke, S. G. (2016). CRC Press; Boca Raton, FL.

Incidental Trainer: A Reference Guide for Training Design, Development and Delivery

Wan, M. (2017). CRC Press; Boca Raton, FL.

Industrial Health

Peterson, J. E. (1991). American Conference of Governmental Hygienists; Cincinnati, OH.

Industrial Mechanics; 3rd Edition

Kemp, A. W. (2012). American Technical; Homewood, IL.

Industrial Safety and Health for Infrastructure Services

Reese, C. D. (2008). CRC Press; Boca Raton, FL.

Industrial-Occupational Hygiene Calculations: A Professional Reference

Stewart, J. H., Herrick, R. F., et al. (1999). Millennium Publishing; Westborough, MA.

Introduction to Fall Protection; 4th Edition

Ellis, J. N. (2011). American Society of Safety Engineers; Des Plaines, IL.

Introduction to Fire Safety Management

Furness, A. & Muckett, M. (2007). Elsevier; Oxford, UK.

Introduction to Risk and Failures

Stamatis, D. H. (2014). CRC Press; Boca Raton, FL.

www.ingramcontent.com/pod-product-compliance
Lightning Source LLC
Chambersburg PA
CBHW081802200326
41597CB00023B/4119